CW00447450

DASH Diet

Cookbook for Beginners 2023

The Ultimate Guide With Healthy, Low-Sodium, High-Potassium, Quick, Easy, and Delicious Recipes to Lower Blood Pressure, Including a 28-Day Meal Prep Plan to Improve Your Health and Lose Weight

Winona Bax

© Copyright 2022 – All rights reserved.

The content contained within this book may not be reproduced, duplicated or transmitted without direct written permission from the author or the publisher.

Under no circumstances will any blame or legal responsibility be held against the publisher, or author, for any damages, reparation, or monetary loss due to the information contained within this book, either directly or indirectly.

Legal Notice:

This book is copyright protected. It is only for personal use. You cannot amend, distribute, sell, use, quote or paraphrase any part, or the content within this book, without the consent of the author or publisher.

Disclaimer Notice:

Please note the information contained within this document is for educational and entertainment purposes only. All effort has been executed to present accurate, up to date, reliable, complete information. No warranties of any kind are declared or implied. Readers acknowledge that the author is not engaged in the rendering of legal, financial, medical or professional advice. The content within this book has been derived from various sources. Please consult a licensed professional before attempting any techniques outlined in this book.

By reading this document, the reader agrees that under no circumstances is the author responsible for any losses, direct or indirect, that are incurred as a result of the use of the information contained within this document, including, but not limited to, errors, omissions or inaccuracies.

Table of Contents

Introduction

Do you want to shed those extra pounds but seem to be struggling? Do you want a natural remedy to lower and maintain your blood pressure levels? Are you looking for a sustainable diet to manage your blood pressure? Do you want to improve your health? If yes, then the DASH diet is perfect for you!

High blood pressure is a silent killer and has become a global concern. Billions worldwide are dealing with high blood pressure; these numbers have doubled in the last couple of decades. High blood pressure or hypertension is a primary risk factor associated with several other chronic health conditions, such as heart disease, stroke, and kidney failure. When it comes to improving your health, you must focus on the diet you consume. Your food choices are vital because some improve your health while others harm it. You are what you eat. One helpful diet known to reduce blood pressure levels is the DASH diet.

The DASH diet is an abbreviation for Dietary Approaches to Stop Hypertension. It was created by the National Heart, Lung, and Blood Institute in the United States. As its name suggests, this dietary protocol is designed to prevent and manage hypertension. Learning to tackle this condition automatically reduces the risk of developing other chronic health problems.

Don't let the word diet fool you. It is not a fad diet that recommends paltry portions or severely restricted eating. Instead, this protocol includes a variety of foods that can be freely consumed, barring a few. Apart from regulating blood pressure, this diet is known to promote weight loss and maintenance, tackle diabetes, and lower the risk of heart diseases and even certain types of cancers. So, you can gain all these benefits by merely changing the diet followed. You will feel healthier and fitter than ever before by following the DASH Diet.

Are you wondering how I know all this? Well, I believe it is time for a little introduction. Hello, my name is Winona Bax, and like you, I used to struggle with high blood pressure. However, I have managed to lower my blood pressure levels and maintain them by shifting to the DASH diet. The countless hours I have spent researching this topic and my personal experience have given me the knowledge needed to regain complete control of my health. Like me, I know even you can improve your health within no time by making healthier dietary choices.

When it comes to following a diet, understanding what it entails is needed. Therefore, the first step is to understand what the DASH diet is all about. Well, you do not have to spend further searching for information about this diet. All the information required about it is given in this book. In this book, you will understand the basics of the DASH diet, its tips, its benefits, and a detailed food list. Once you are armed with this information, you will be introduced to various DASH diet-friendly recipes. The recipes are divided into different categories for convenience and ease of use. This book will act as your guide for every step, from breakfast, lunch, and dinner recipes to salads, sauces, and sides, vegetarian and vegan options, and appetizers and snacks. We will also introduce you to a sample four-week meal plan to start with this diet.

Well, are you eager to learn more about the DASH diet? Do you want to regain control of your health? If yes, it's time to get started.

Chapter 1: About the DASH Diet

fundamental aspect of ensuring your overall health is the diet you follow. When you ink of a diet, chances are you visualize paltry portions or extremely limited food choices. owever, following a well-balanced diet is needed to improve your health and reduce the sk of certain diseases and illnesses.

ne health problem that has become a global crisis is hypertension or high blood pressure. here are billions across the globe suffering from this condition. It is often dubbed a silent ller because it has no apparent symptoms or signs. However, its ramifications are critical. or instance, high blood pressure is the primary marker for chronic health conditions such strokes and cardiovascular disorders. Do not get worried reading through all this. The od news is that your diet is within your control. You can always change even if you are not ting healthily right now. This is where the DASH diet steps into the picture.

What Is the DASH Diet?

ASH diet stands for Dietary Approaches to Stop Hypertension. It was created by the nited States National Heart, Lung, and Blood Institute. As its name suggests, this diet was eated solely to reduce hypertension and its risks. Before understanding what it means, essential to understand what blood pressure means. The force on the blood vessels and gans as the blood passes through them is known as blood pressure. It is counted in terms systolic and diastolic pressure. The pressure within the blood vessels when the heart beats systolic pressure. Diastolic pressure is the one that exists in the blood vessels in between artbeats or when the heart is at rest. Typically, the systolic and diastolic pressures must be 0 over 80. To those with hypertension, the blood pressure reading is usually more than 140 er 90.

e DASH diet effectively regulates high blood pressure because it drastically limits salt or dium intake. The daily sodium intake is restricted to 2,300 mg and is in synchronization th the dietary guidelines issued by most governments. This is a predominantly plant-based t but also includes sufficient quantities of animal-based foods. This diet is well-rounded, m wholesome fruits and vegetables to whole grains, lean proteins, nuts and seeds, and althy fats. Unlike a typical Western diet, it is not rich in processed and prepackaged foods, healthy fats, harmful carbs, added sugars, and excess sodium. This is one of the reasons why DASH diet successfully reduces blood pressure levels in comparison to other diets.

Benefits of the DASH Diet

Even though making a dietary change does not sound like much, it is a significant change for your body and mind. Focusing on all the benefits automatically increases the motivation to stick to it whenever you need to change. Now that you understand what this diet means and how it works, let's look at its benefits.

Reduces Blood Pressure

As mentioned, to those with hypertension, the blood pressure readings are above 140 over 90. These numbers stand for the systolic and diastolic pressures, respectively. This diet helps lower systolic and diastolic pressures (Sacks et al., 1999). By following the low-salt DASH diet, you can regulate your blood pressure levels.

Promotes Weight Loss

Weight loss is usually recommended for those with high blood pressure. This is because the greater the body weight, the higher the blood pressure. Therefore, losing weight helps regulate your blood pressure. A wonderful thing about the DASH diet is it helps promote weight loss (Ndanuko et al., 2016). This, in turn, helps reduce blood pressure and maintain

Other Health Benefits

Apart from the benefits mentioned above, this diet offers other health benefits. It's believed that the DASH diet helps reduce the risk of certain cancers, such as breast and colorectal cancer (Onvani et al., 2015). This diet helps reduce the risk of metabolic syndrome (Saneei et al., 2014). This diet also reduces the risk of type 2 diabetes (Hinderliter et al., 2011). The consumption of healthy foods and the restriction of unhealthy ones are known to improve heart health and reduce the risk of cardiovascular disorders too (Salehi-Abargouei et al., 2013). So shifting to the DASH diet is not only good for regulating hypertension but for improving your overall health as well!

Food List

Unlike most diets, the DASH diet is not restrictive by any means. It includes all the differe food groups. The only consideration is to ensure that you do not consume excess sodium. Apart from this, you must be mindful of your processed and prepackaged food intake. As you go through the food list, one thing will become evident; the DASH diet increases the consumption of wholesome and nutritious ingredients while limiting unhealthy ones.

Foods to Eat

hen making a dietary change, it is important to focus on all the different types of foods
u can eat instead of worrying about the ones you cannot or should not eat. Doing this
ates a positive mindset that makes it easier to stick to the diet. Here is a list of foods you
n consume while following the DASH diet.

Whole Grains

hole grains are an excellent source of complex carbohydrates your body requires
function effectively and efficiently. They are also rich in dietary fiber, antioxidants,
complex vitamins, iron, and magnesium. As per the DASH diet, you can consume six to
ht servings of whole grains daily. Whether oatmeal for breakfast or whole wheat pasta for
ner, these are excellent means to incorporate whole grains into your diet. When selecting
ole grains, you must look for unprocessed ones instead of processed and polished variants.
nile purchasing bread or pasta, opt for ones made with whole grains.

Vegetables

getables are one of the healthiest categories of ingredients that you can incorporate into
diet. Vegetables are incredibly healthy and contain most of the nutrients your body
uires. You can consume five to six servings of vegetables daily on this diet. You can easily
lude vegetables in daily meals, from salads and soups to side dishes. Add vegetables of
erent colors to ensure your body gets all the nutrients it needs. There are no restrictions,
n root vegetables to cruciferous vegetables, leafy greens, and nightshades.

Fruits

can consume all fruits while following the DASH diet. This diet recommends
suming around four to five servings of fruits daily. Don't fear the natural sugars present
ruits. They are not harmful. Instead, the only sugars to be avoided are artificial sweeteners
all added sugars. Whether it is snacks, desserts, or smoothies, incorporate different types
uits into your daily meals. There are no restrictions, from apples, plums, and tropical
ts to citrus fruits and berries.

Dairy Products

iding high levels of saturated fats is not only healthy but is recommended by the DASH
. Instead of full-fat dairy products, you can opt for low-fat or fat-free ones. Whether it is

fat-free milk, low-fat cheese, or fat-free yogurt, feel free to include them in your daily diet. However, ensure your daily consumption is restricted to two to three servings.

Lean Proteins

Even though the DASH diet is predominantly plant-based, it includes a healthy dose of lea protein. You can consume up to 6 oz of lean protein daily. It probably doesn't seem like a l but you can consume plenty of skinless poultry, eggs, fatty fish, and low-fat cuts of red mea within this quota. You can also include tofu and tempeh to obtain the protein your body requires.

Fats and Oils

Paying attention to the fats and oils you cook with is essential not just when you are following the DASH diet but any other diet as well. As mentioned, all fats are not the sam Whenever you are cooking, opt for monounsaturated fats. Some common examples inclu olive oil, safflower oil, avocado oil, and canola oil. Ensure your consumption of fats and oi restricted to two to three servings per day.

Nuts, Seeds, and Beans

Ensure you consume nuts, seeds, beans, and different legumes around four to five times pe week. These foods are an excellent source of heart-healthy dietary fats and fiber. They alsc contain helpful nutrients, vitamins, and minerals. Since these foods are naturally rich in calories, regulate their intake. Some common examples of nuts, seeds, and legumes you ca consume are almonds, walnuts, flaxseeds, sunflower seeds, kidney beans, and lentils.

Foods to Avoid

The DASH diet is designed to automatically eliminate or severely limit the consumption certain foods that increase blood pressure levels and harm the heart's health. In the previo section, we introduced you to all the foods you can consume while following this diet. N let's look at the categories of foods that must be avoided while following this eating patte

Any ingredient that is rich in sodium is harmful to your overall health and functioning. Reducing dietary salt helps reduce the risk of hypertension, strokes, and cardiovascular disorders. Some everyday items you must avoid are processed meats, prepackaged and processed foods, and fast food. Apart from this, it severely reduces the consumption of tab salt.

ats are an essential part of a healthy diet. However, all fats are not the same. Some improve our health, while others harm it. One such category of fats you need to avoid is saturated its. Reducing the intake of foods rich in saturated fats helps improve your cardiovascular ealth and regulates blood pressure. Some common types of items that you need to avoid are hole milk, cheese, full-fat cream and butter, full-fat yogurt, poultry with skin, and fatty cuts f meat.

ny food item that has added sugar must be avoided. Whether it is adding a cube of sugar your daily cup of coffee or packaged foods, sugar is your enemy. So some common tegories of foods you need to avoid are food products with added sugar, fast food and junk od, and table sugar. You can consume desserts in moderation. Yes, that's right. You don't ve to give up on sweet treats for the sake of following this diet. Instead, you need to make ealthier choices. You will be introduced to various DASH diet-friendly dessert recipes later this book.

egulation is an essential aspect of the DASH diet or any other diet. Just because you are owed to consume a specific ingredient category does not mean you go overboard. This et recommends limited consumption of red meats without any fat. However, loading up excess red meat is detrimental to your health, not just hypertension. As mentioned, this et is not restrictive by any means. It simply restricts the consumption of unhealthy foods.

Shopping List

eping the considerations mentioned above in mind, here is a sample shopping list you can low to stick to this diet. As a rule of thumb, ensure you have a list before going grocery opping. To make things easier, go through the recipes in this book and the sample meal in. This ensures your pantry is stocked with the needed ingredients. Once these things are place, cooking becomes easy. Also, this is just an example of how your shopping list on the SH diet must look like. It can be customized and changed as per your requirements. An portant factor is to ensure you include all the food groups mentioned here.

Whole Grains

whole wheat bread and pasta

oatmeal

brown rice

processed whole grains such as unsalted pretzels, popcorn, rolls, and English muffins

Vegetables

- broccoli
- brussels sprouts
- potatoes
- spinach
- amaranth
- carrots
- collard greens
- green peas
- green beans
- lettuce
- arugula
- Swiss chard
- daikon
- fennel
- radish
- beets
- onions
- sweet potatoes
- squashes and gourds

Fruits

- apples
- bananas
- grapes
- oranges
- peaches
- strawberries
- dates
- grapefruit
- tangerine
- all berries

Low-Fat Dairy Products

low-fat cheese

fat-free milk

plant-based milk and yogurt

fat-free yogurt

Meat, Fish, and Poultry

skinless chicken and turkey

eggs

lean cuts of lamb, beef, and pork

fatty fish such as salmon, herring, cod, sardines, mackerel, and trout

Fats and Oils

olive oil

avocado oil

safflower oil

Nuts, Seeds, and Beans

almonds

walnuts

cashew nuts

macadamia

hazelnuts

pecans

chia seeds

flaxseeds

hempseeds

sesame seeds

cannellini beans

black beans

chickpeas

- green peas
- split peas
- soybeans
- edamame
- kidney beans
- sunflower seeds

Tips to Reduce Sodium Intake

Excess sodium intake is the primary cause of high blood pressure. So cutting it out of your diet is important to regulate hypertension. While following the DASH diet, your sodium intake will reduce. That said, here are some additional tips that can be used to further curtail your sodium intake.

Instead of using salt as the primary flavoring while cooking, opt for other seasonings, herb aromatics, and citrus to enhance the flavor profile of any meal you cook.

Make it a point to track your daily sodium intake without failing. This ensures you're not exceeding the needed sodium intake. These days, a variety of apps can be used to do this.

While purchasing any packaged or processed foods, carefully read through the nutrition label. Check the sodium content as per the serving sizes and portions. This is especially true for frozen and canned foods. For instance, foods packed with saline, sodium, or broth must be avoided. If you are using canned vegetables or beans, drain and rinse them before cook or eating.

If eating out, check if your meals can be cooked without salt. Similarly, some common sau and condiments that must be avoided because of their high sodium content are soy sauce, miso, most Asian sauces, and tomato sauce. Also, anything smoked, cured, brined, pickled, o barbecued should be avoided.

Weight Loss Tips

Even though the DASH diet is not restrictive, understand that it is not a license to overea or binge. If you strictly follow the protocols suggested by it, you will experience weight loss. However, if weight loss is also your priority, you will need to be mindful of your food choices. Apart from this, you should also closely observe the calories you consume. For weight loss, a calorie deficit is needed. This condition occurs when your calorie consumption is lower than your calorie expenditure. The simplest way to maintain a calo deficit is to reduce your calorie consumption or increase calorie expenditure. Ideally, ensu you stick to the 2,000 calories per day limit, and you will notice weight loss within a cou weeks.

nother reason this diet promotes weight loss is due to sodium restriction. Reducing
odium consumption results in the loss of water weight. To further speed up the process,
nsure you do not consume more sodium than the diet prescribes. Instead of using salt, opt
or herbs, salt-free seasonings, spices, and other aromatics to flavor your meals. Similarly, avoid
lting the food after it is cooked.

you follow the recipes given in this book, you can dig into healthy and delicious meals
ithout worrying about extra salt. Another suggestion is that you can use it to practice
indful eating. It means you must eat only when hungry and stop when satiated. Also, don't
t just because you should; instead, eat when hungry. While eating, pay attention to your
od and focus only on it without getting distracted.

nother great way to not just speed up weight loss but improve your overall health is by
ercising regularly. Exercise also increases caloric expenditure resulting in a natural calorie
ficit. Ensure that you exercise for at least 20 minutes daily. If not, aim for around 3–4
urs of exercise per week. That's about it. A little movement is all it takes to improve your
alth.

mentioned, you need to be mindful of your food choices. Nuts, seeds, and legumes are
althy but are rich in calories. Eating too many of these ingredients will automatically
crease your calorie consumption. Similarly, filling up on desserts, even if they are DASH
t-friendly, is not a good idea. Ensure you focus on wholesome grains, vegetables, lean
oteins, and fruits before moving on to other food groups. This ensures your body gets its
ily dose of nutrients without compromising health.

you are used to snacking regularly, you must make healthier choices. There are different
althy snacking recipes and ideas given in this book. Go through them and stock up
them. Instead of digging into junk food, replace it with fresh and wholesome foods.
llowing this diet will become extremely simple with a little planning and preparation.

Chapter 2: DASH Diet Breakfast Recipes

Oat and Nut Breakfast Bars

Time: 35 minutes

Serving Size: 12

Prep Time: 5 minutes

Cook Time: 30 minutes

Nutrition Facts Per Serving (1 bar):

Calories: 169

Fat: 5 g

Total Carbohydrate: 26 g

Protein: 5 g

Sodium: 81 mg

Ingredients:

- 1 ¼ cups old-fashioned rolled oats
- ¼ cup fat-free dry milk
- ¼ cup sliced, toasted almonds or pecans
- ¼ cup raisins
- ½ cup dark honey
- ½ tbsp olive oil
- ¼ cup soy flour
- ¼ cup toasted wheat germ
- ¼ cup chopped dried apples
- ¼ tsp salt
- ¼ cup natural peanut butter, unsalted
- 1 tsp vanilla extract

Directions:

1. Preheat your oven to 325 °F. Grease a small baking dish (about 8 inches) with cooking spray.
2. Combine honey, oil, and peanut butter in a saucepan and cook the mixture over medium heat. Stir frequently until the mixture just melts and is smooth. Make sure you do not boil the mixture.
3. Turn off the heat. Add vanilla and stir. Cool until it is warm.
4. Add oats, dry milk, nuts, raisins, soy flour, wheat germ, apples, and salt into another bowl. Mix well. Pour the warm honey mixture and mix well.
5. Transfer the mixture to the prepared baking dish. Spread it evenly, pressing it you spread, and place it in the oven.
6. Set the timer for about 15–20 minutes or until the edges are getting light brown.
7. Remove from the oven and cool on a wire rack for 10 minutes.
8. Slice into 12 equal bars. Let it cool before serving. Leftover bars can be placed in an airtight container in the refrigerator until use.

Cranberry Orange Muffins

Time: 32 minutes

Serving Size: 8

Prep Time: 8–10 minutes

Cook Time: 22 minutes

Nutritional Facts Per Serving (1 muffin):

lories: 165

t: 5 g

tal Carbohydrate: 27 g

otein: 4 g

dium: 188 mg

gredients:

½ cup nonfat plain Greek yogurt

1 egg

2 tbsp canola oil

1 grated tbsp of orange zest

½ cup plus 6 tbsp all-purpose flour

½ tsp baking powder

2 tbsp flaxseed meal

½ tsp baking soda

¼ tsp ground cinnamon

½ cup sugar

2 tbsp brown sugar

1 tbsp orange juice concentrate

1 tsp vanilla extract

¼ tsp salt

¾ cup cranberries, fresh or frozen

ections:

Prepare the oven by preheating it to 350 °F. Grease muffin cups or a muffin tin with cooking spray or butter. Line the cups with disposable liners as well.

Add the dry ingredients (i.e., sugar, yogurt, oil, egg, orange juice, vanilla, and orange zest) into a bowl and stir. Add flour, flaxseed, baking powder, baking soda, cinnamon, and salt into another bowl and mix well.

Combine the dry ingredients and wet ingredients. Beat with an electric mixer on low speed until well combined. Add cranberries and fold gently.

4. Pour the batter into the prepared muffin tins, up to three fourths.

5. Place the muffin tin in the oven and set the timer for about 22 minutes or until the top is golden brown.

Nut and Berry Parfait

Time: 5 minutes

Serving Size: 2

Prep Time: 5 minutes

Cook Time: none

Nutritional Facts Per Serving (1 glass):

Calories: 378

Fat: 15 g

Total Carbohydrate: 35 g

Protein: 20 g

Sodium: 83 mg

Ingredients:

- 2 cups nonfat plain Greek yogurt
- ½ cup fresh or frozen blueberries
- ½ cup fresh or frozen raspberries
- 4 tsp honey
- ½ cup sliced almonds, toasted

Directions:

1. Take two parfait glasses. Place a layer of each—yogurt, berries, and almonds. Repeat the layers once again with the remaining ingredients.

2. Drizzle 2 tsp of honey in each glass and serve.

Summer Skillet Vegetable and Egg Scramble

Time: 30 minutes

Serving Size: 3

Prep Time: 10 minutes

Cook Time: 20 minutes

Nutritional Facts Per Serving (1 ½ cups):

Calories: 254

Fat: 14.2 g

Total Carbohydrate: 19.7 g

Protein: 12.4 g

Sodium: 415 mg

Ingredients:

- 1 tbsp olive oil
- 2 cups thinly sliced mixed vegetables (a mixture of bell peppers, mushrooms, and zucchini)
- ½ tsp minced fresh herbs of your choice
- 1 cup packed baby spinach or kale
- 6 oz baby potatoes, thinly sliced
- 1 ½ cups scallion, thinly sliced (keep the whites and greens separate)
- 3 large eggs, lightly beaten
- ¼ tsp salt

Directions:

1. Pour oil into a nonstick pan and let it heat over medium heat. When the oil is hot, add the potatoes and stir, then cover the pan. Cook until potatoes are slightly tender, stirring regularly.
2. Stir in the mixed vegetables and whites of the scallions and cook with the lid on until the vegetables are light brown.
3. Add fresh herbs and mix well.
4. Push the vegetables to the sides of the pan. Turn down the heat to medium-low. Crack eggs into the center of the pan. Also, add the scallion greens over the eggs. Stir the eggs until they are sof[t] cooked.
5. Next, add the spinach and mix it with [the] eggs. Now mix the egg mixture and th[e] vegetables and turn the heat off.
6. Add salt and stir. Serve hot.

Vegan Sweet Potato Waffles

Time: 11 minutes

Serving Size: 2

Prep Time: 3 minutes

Cook Time: 8 minutes

Nutritional Facts Per Serving (1 waff[le):

Calories: 263

Fat: 7 g

Total Carbohydrate: 41.6 g

Protein: 9.41 g

Sodium: 57 mg

Ingredients:

- ¾ cup oat flour
- ½ tsp baking powder
- ½ tbsp chia egg or flax egg
- ½ cup nondairy milk of your choice
- ½ tsp ground cinnamon
- a tiny pinch of salt

- 3 tbsp cooked mashed sweet potatoes
- ½ tbsp maple syrup (optional)

Directions:

1. To make a chia or flax egg, combine chia or flaxseeds and 1 ½ tbsp of water in a bowl. Place the bowl in the refrigerator for 15 minutes. It will become gel-like.

2. Add baking powder, cinnamon, salt, and oat flour in a bowl and stir.

3. Add flax egg, milk, sweet potato, and maple syrup into a bowl and whisk until smooth. Add the sweet potato mixture into the bowl of dry ingredients and fold until well combined. You can use sweet potato puree or roast and mash sweet potato for sweet potato mash.

. Set up your waffle iron and preheat it according to the manufacturer's instructions. Grease it a bit with some cooking spray or butter.

. Scoop half the batter into the waffle iron and spread it. Close the lid and let it cook for 3–4 minutes or until cooked to your satisfaction. Take out the waffle and serve it with toppings of your choice.

. Make the remaining waffle similarly.

Chapter 3: Lunch Recipes

Chimichurri Noodle Bowls

Time: 28 minutes

Serving Size: 2

Prep Time: 8 minutes

Cook Time: 20 minutes

Nutritional Facts Per Serving (3 cups or 1 bowl):

Calories: 377

Fat: 19.9 g

Total Carbohydrate: 28.1 g

Protein: 24.8 g

Sodium: 376 mg

Ingredients:

- chimichurri sauce
- 1 cup fresh flat-leaf parsley
- 1 ½ tbsp lemon juice
- ¼ tsp crushed red pepper
- 2–3 garlic cloves, sliced
- ½ tbsp chopped fresh oregano or ½ tsp dried oregano
- ¼ tsp salt
- ¼ cup extra-virgin olive oil
- 2 oz whole-grain spaghetti
- 6 oz cooked shrimp, peeled
- 4 cups zucchini noodles
- ⅛ cup crumbled feta cheese

Directions:

1. Boil the spaghetti following the directions given on the package.
2. To make the chimichurri sauce, blend parsley, lemon juice, red pepper, garlic, oregano, and salt in a blender until smooth. With the blender machine running, pour oil in a thin drizzle. Continue blending until smooth and well combined.
3. Make zucchini noodles of the zucchini using a spiralizer or julienne peeler. Combine shrimp, feta, spaghetti, and zucchini noodles in a bowl. Add chimichurri sauce and toss well.
4. Divide the noodles into two bowls and serve.

Buffalo Chicken Salad Wrap

Time: 22 minutes

Serving Size: 2

Prep Time: 10 minutes

Cook Time: 10–12 minutes

Nutritional Facts Per Serving (½ wrap)

Calories: 300

Fat: 8 g

Total Carbohydrate: 26 g

Protein: 31 g

Sodium: 367 mg

Ingredients:

- 1.5–2 oz chicken breasts
- 2 tbsp white wine vinegar

1 stalk celery, diced

¼ cup chopped yellow onion

2 oz spinach, thinly sliced

1 whole chipotle pepper

2 tbsp low-calorie mayonnaise

1 carrot, cut into matchsticks

¼ cup rutabaga, thinly sliced

2 whole-grain tortillas (6 inches each)

rections:

You can use leftover rotisserie chicken instead of chicken breasts.

If you use chicken breasts, roast the chicken in an oven or cook on a grill until it is cooked well inside (5–6 minutes on each side). Chop the chicken into cubes.

Add chipotle pepper, mayonnaise, and vinegar to blend until smooth.

Add the blended mixture, chicken, celery, onion, carrot, and rutabaga into a bowl and mix well.

Spread the mixture equally over the tortillas. Divide the spinach among the tortillas. Wrap and place with its seam side down. Cut into two halves and serve.

Quinoa Egg Salad Wrap

1e: 25 minutes

ving Size: 2

p Time: 10 minutes

ok Time: 15 minutes

ritional Facts Per Serving (½ wrap):

Calories: 233

Fat: 9 g

Total Carbohydrate: 32 g

Protein: 17 g

Sodium: 376 mg

Ingredients:

- 1 tbsp mayonnaise
- 3.5 oz canned or cooked red kidney beans, drained, rinsed
- 0.9 oz mature cheddar cheese, grated
- pepper to taste & 1 tbsp finely chopped scallions or green onions
- 1 large tortilla
- ¼ cup cooked quinoa
- 1 tbsp Greek yogurt & ⅔ tsp Dijon mustard
- ½ tbsp chia seeds
- 1 tbsp finely chopped parsley
- fine sea salt to taste
- 2 large eggs, hard boiled, peeled, finely chopped

Directions:

1. Add quinoa, yogurt, mustard, chia seeds, parsley, salt, eggs, pepper, mayonnaise, kidney beans, cheese, and scallions into a bowl and mix well.

2. Place this mixture on the tortilla. Fold like a burrito. Cut into two halves and serve. You can also serve it cold. If you want to serve cold, keep the wrap covered in paper in the refrigerator until use. Then unwrap, cut into two and serve.

Tuna Pita Pockets

Time: 5 minutes

Serving Size: 3

Prep Time: 5 minutes

Cook Time: none

Nutritional Facts Per Serving (1 stuffed pita pocket):

Calories: 209

Fat: 5 g

Total Carbohydrate: 23 g

Protein: 18 g

Sodium: 378 mg

Ingredients:

- ¾ cup shredded romaine lettuce
- ¼ cup finely chopped green bell pepper
- ¼ cup finely chopped broccoli
- 1 can (6 oz) low-salt white tuna in water, drained
- 1 ½ whole wheat pita pockets (cut the whole one into two halves)
- 1 diced tomato
- ¼ cup shredded carrots
- ⅛ cup finely chopped onion
- ¼ cup low-fat ranch dressing

Directions:

1. Combine the vegetables in a bowl.
2. Combine tuna and ranch dressing in another bowl.
3. Now combine the ingredients of both bowls.
4. Fill the pita pockets with the tuna and vegetable mixture before serving.

Chicken Burritos

Time: 30 minutes

Serving Size: 2

Prep Time: 10 minutes

Cook Time: 20 minutes

Nutritional Facts Per Serving (1 burrito):

Calories: 286

Fat: 6 g

Total Carbohydrate: 38 g

Protein: 20 g

Sodium: 382 mg

Ingredients:

- ½ tsp oil
- ½ jalapeño pepper, deseeded, chopped
- ½ yellow onion, chopped
- 1 cup grape tomatoes
- 4 oz cooked chicken breast, shredded
- ¼ cup canned or cooked unsalted black beans, drained, rinsed
- ½ red bell pepper, chopped
- 1 rib celery, chopped & 1 tbsp cumin seeds
- 1 clove garlic, chopped
- 2 whole wheat tortillas (10 inches each)
- 1 cup green cabbage, shredded

Directions:

1. Pour oil into a skillet and let it heat ov medium-high heat. When the oil is ho add cumin seeds. When the cumin see crackle, add bell pepper, garlic, onion, celery and mix well.
2. Stir often until the vegetables are sligh

tender. Stir in the tomatoes and oregano and cook for a few minutes until the tomatoes start bursting at the skin. Turn off the heat. Blend the mixture until smooth or the preferred consistency.

3. To assemble, spread an equal quantity of chicken on the tortillas. Spread an equal quantity of beans and cabbage over the chicken. Drizzle sauce on top and fold like a burrito.

4. Serve.

Add beef, onion, and pepper and stir. As you stir, break the meat into crumbles. When the meat is brown, discard excess fat from the pan.

2. Place the pan back over medium heat. Stir in the tomato soup. Boil gently on low heat until the mixture is almost dry.

3. Serve over buns.

Sloppy Joes

Time: 20 minutes

Serving Size: 3

Prep Time: 5 minutes

Cook Time: 12–15 minutes

Nutritional Facts Per Serving (1 sandwich):

Calories: 251

Fat: 9 g

Total Carbohydrate: 28 g

Protein: 19 g

Sodium: 203 mg

Ingredients:

½ lb 90% lean ground beef

½ cup chopped onions

3 whole wheat hamburger buns, split

½ cup chopped green bell pepper

1 cup low-sodium tomato soup, undiluted

Directions:

Heat a nonstick pan over medium heat.

Chapter 4: Dinner Recipes

Chicken Quesadillas

Time: 30 minutes

Serving Size: 3

Prep Time: 10 minutes

Cook Time: 18–20 minutes

Nutritional Facts Per Serving (2 halves):

Calories: 298

Fat: 10 g

Total Carbohydrate: 25 g

Protein: 27 g

Sodium: 524 mg

Ingredients:

- 2 skinless, boneless chicken breasts (4 oz each), cut into cubes
- ¼ cup smoky or hot salsa
- ½ cup chopped fresh cilantro
- ½ cup shredded low-fat cheddar cheese
- ½ cup chopped onions
- ½ cup chopped fresh tomatoes
- 3 whole wheat tortillas (8 inches each)

Directions:

1. Preheat the oven to 425 °F. Prepare a baking sheet by greasing it with cooking spray.
2. Cook chicken and onions in a nonstick pan. When the chicken is well cooked, turn off the heat. Add tomatoes, salsa, and cilantro and stir.
3. To make quesadillas, place tortillas on your countertop and brush their edges with some water. Divide the chicken mixture equally and place it on each of the tortillas. Spread it all over the tortilla except around the edges, where you hav brushed the water.
4. Sprinkle cheddar cheese on top of the tortillas. Make a semicircle from each tortilla by folding it in half over itself.
5. Press the edges together to seal. Place the folded tortillas on the baking sheet. Spray some cooking spray on top of the tortillas. Place the baking sheet in the oven and set the timer for 6–8 minutes until a little crisp and brown.
6. Cut each into two halves and serve.

Chicken Quinoa Bowl With Olives and Cucumber

Time: 28 minutes

Serving Size: 2

Prep Time: 10 minutes

Cook Time: 15–18 minutes

Nutritional Facts Per Serving (1 bowl

Calories: 519

Fat: 26.9 g

Total Carbohydrate: 31.2 g

Protein: 34.1 g

Sodium: 683.5 mg

Ingredients:

½ lb boneless, skinless chicken breasts, trimmed

⅛ tsp pepper

⅛ cup slivered almonds

½ small clove garlic, crushed

¼ tsp ground cumin

⅛ tsp salt

½ tsp paprika

⅛ tsp crushed red pepper

⅛ cup pitted kalamata olives, chopped

½ cup diced cucumber

1 tbsp finely chopped fresh parsley

½ jar (from a 7-oz jar) of roasted red peppers, rinsed

2 tbsp extra-virgin olive oil, divided

1 cup cooked quinoa

⅛ cup finely chopped onion

⅛ cup crumbled feta cheese

Directions:

Place the rack in the upper third position in the oven. Set the oven to broil mode and preheat to high heat. Prepare a trimmed baking sheet by lining it with foil.

Season the chicken with salt and pepper and lay it on the baking sheet. Place it in the oven and broil for 7–8 minutes on each side or until the internal temperature of the chicken in the meatiest part shows 165 °F on the meat thermometer.

Take out the baking sheet and let the chicken cool for a while. Cut the chicken into slices, or you can even shred it.

4. In the meantime, blend roasted pepper, 1 tbsp oil, almonds, garlic, and spices in the mini food processor until nearly smooth.

5. Add quinoa, 1 tbsp oil, onion, and olives into a bowl and mix well.

6. To assemble, distribute equally the quinoa mixture into two bowls. Distribute the cucumber and chicken equally and place them over the quinoa. Drizzle red pepper sauce on top. Garnish with feta and parsley and serve.

Fried Rice

Time: 17 minutes

Serving Size: 2

Prep Time: 5 minutes

Cook Time: 10–12 minutes

Nutritional Facts Per Serving (½ recipe):

Calories: 279

Fat: 16 g

Total Carbohydrate: 31 g

Protein: 6 g

Sodium: 116 mg

Ingredients:

- 1 cup cooked brown rice
- 2 green onions, chopped
- ¼ cup finely chopped green bell pepper
- 1 small egg, beaten
- ½ tbsp sesame oil
- 1 ½ tbsp peanut oil
- 1 carrot, finely chopped
- ¼ cup frozen peas, thawed

- 1 tbsp low-sodium soy sauce
- 2 tbsp chopped parsley

Directions:

1. Pour oil into a wok and let it heat over medium heat. When the oil is hot, add rice and cook for a few minutes until golden brown. Stir on and off.

2. Stir in the vegetables and cook until the vegetables are crisp as well as tender. Push the rice and vegetables to the sides of the wok and pour the beaten egg in the center. Stir often until the egg is scrambled.

3. Now mix the rice and eggs thoroughly. Add soy sauce and mix well. Drizzle sesame oil on top. Garnish with parsley and serve.

Grilled Portobello Mushroom Burgers

Time: 1 hour 15 minutes

Serving Size: 2

Prep Time: 1 hour 5 minutes (marinating time included)

Cook Time: 10 minutes

Nutritional Facts Per Serving (1 burger):

Calories: 301

Fat: 9 g

Total Carbohydrate: 45 g

Protein: 10 g

Sodium: 163 mg

Ingredients:

- 2 large portobello mushroom caps (abo 5 inches each), cleaned, stem discarded
- ¼ cup water
- 2 ½ tbsp balsamic vinegar
- ½ tbsp sugar
- a pinch of cayenne pepper
- 2 whole wheat buns, split, toasted
- 2 slices red onion
- ½ clove garlic, minced
- 1 tbsp olive oil
- 2 slices tomato
- 1 Bibb lettuce, halved

Directions:

1. Place mushrooms in a glass dish with t stem side facing up.

2. For the marinade, combine vinegar, su cayenne pepper, water, garlic, and oil in a bowl. Pour the marinade over the mushrooms. Cover the bowl and chill an hour. Turn the mushrooms once aft 30 minutes of marinating.

3. Remove the mushroom from the marinating liquid. Grill or broil the mushrooms for about 5 minutes on each side. Brush the marinade over the mushrooms while grilling.

4. To assemble, place a mushroom, a tom slice, an onion slice, and one piece of lettuce on the bottom half of each bur Cover the burger with the top half of buns.

5. Serve right away.

Black Bean Wrap

Time: 15 minutes

Serving Size: 3

Prep Time: 10 minutes

Cook Time: 5 minutes

Nutritional Facts Per Serving (1 wrap):

Calories: 341

Fat: 9 g

Total Carbohydrate: 50 g

Protein: 15 g

Sodium: 633 mg

Ingredients:

¾ cup frozen corn kernels, thawed

1 tbsp chopped green chili peppers, deseeded

½ tomato, diced

3 fat-free, whole-grain tortilla wraps (10 inches each)

6 tbsp salsa

¾ cup cooked or canned low-sodium or unsalted black beans, rinsed and drained

a handful of chopped fresh cilantro

2 green onions, sliced

½ tbsp chopped garlic

6 tbsp shredded cheddar cheese

Directions:

1. Place corn, black beans, chili peppers, tomato, cilantro, onion, and garlic in a microwave-safe container and let it heat on high for about a minute.

2. Warm the tortillas following the directions on the package.

3. To assemble, spread about ½ cup of beans in the center of each tortilla.

4. Scatter 2 tbsp of cheese on each tortilla.

5. Spread 2 tbsp of salsa on each.

6. Fold like a burrito and serve.

Chickpea Pasta With Mushrooms and Kale

Time: 33 minutes

Serving Size: 2

Prep Time: 5–8 minutes

Cook Time: 25 minutes

Nutritional Facts Per Serving (1 ½ cups):

Calories: 340

Fat: 18 g

Total Carbohydrate: 38 g

Protein: 17 g

Sodium: 366 mg

Ingredients:

- 4 oz chickpea rotini or penne pasta
- 1 large clove garlic, sliced
- 4 cups chopped kale
- ¼ tsp dried thyme
- grated Parmesan cheese to serve (optional)
- 2 tbsp extra-virgin olive oil
- crushed red pepper to taste
- 4 oz cremini mushrooms, quartered
- ¼ tsp salt

Directions:

1. Follow the directions given on the

package of the pasta and cook it accordingly. Retain about ½ cup of the cooked pasta water and discard the rest.

2. Pour oil into a pan and let it heat over medium heat. When the oil is hot, stir in the garlic and cook for a few seconds until you get a nice aroma. Next, mix it well with mushrooms, kale, red pepper, and salt.

3. When the vegetables are soft, add pasta and the retained water and mix well. Heat thoroughly.

4. Garnish with Parmesan and serve.

Chapter 5: Salad Recipes

Beet and Orange Salad

Time: 1 hour 8 minutes

Serving Size: 2

Prep Time: 8 minutes

Cook Time: 60 minutes

Nutritional Facts Per Serving (½ recipe):

Calories: 118

Fat: 2 g

Total Carbohydrate: 22 g

Protein: 3 g

Sodium: 135 mg

Ingredients:

2 cups baby beets, trimmed, rinsed

½ cup thinly sliced beet greens

¾ cup Napa cabbage

juice of ½ orange & zest of ½ orange

¾ tsp olive oil plus extra to brush the beets

¼ cup chopped celery

¼ cup chopped yellow onion

½ orange, peeled, separated into segments

pepper to taste

Directions:

1. Preheat the oven to 400 °F. Brush oil over the beets and wrap them in foil. Place the foil packet in the oven and roast until they are cooked through, about 45–60 minutes.

2. Take out the packet and unwrap it. Let the beets cool for a while. Peel off the skin and cut it into slices. Place beets, orange segments, greens, celery, onion, cabbage, orange juice, orange zest, pepper, and oil into a bowl and toss well.

3. Serve onto two plates.

Cucumber and Pineapple Salad

Time: 15 minutes

Serving Size: 2

Prep Time: 10 minutes

Cook Time: 5 minutes

Nutritional Facts Per Serving (1 ½ cups):

Calories: 129

Fat: 1 g

Total Carbohydrate: 28 g

Protein: 2 g

Sodium: 102 mg

Ingredients:

- 2 tbsp sugar
- 1 tbsp water
- ½ cucumber, peeled, thinly sliced
- ½ small red onion, thinly sliced
- ½ tbsp toasted sesame seeds
- ⅓ cup rice wine vinegar
- ½ cup canned, unsweetened pineapple chunks

- ½ carrot, julienned
- 2 cups torn salad greens

Directions:

1. Combine sugar, water, and vinegar in a heavy saucepan and place the saucepan over medium heat. Stir until the sugar melts and the liquid in the saucepan is about ¼ cup. Turn off the heat and pour it into a bowl. Transfer the bowl to the refrigerator and let it cool down.

2. Now add the vegetables and pineapple into the bowl of cooled liquid. Mix well.

3. Distribute the salad greens onto two serving plates. Distribute the vegetable and pineapple salad equally and place them over the greens. Garnish with sesame seeds and serve.

Chicken Salad

Time: 20 minutes

Serving Size: 2

Prep Time: 10 minutes

Cook Time: 10 minutes

Nutritional Facts Per Serving (½ recipe):

Calories: 237

Fat: 9 g

Total Carbohydrate: 12 g

Protein: 27 g

Sodium: 199 mg

Ingredients:

- Dressing
- ¼ cup red wine vinegar
- ½ tbsp extra-virgin olive oil
- ½ tbsp finely chopped celery
- 2 garlic cloves, minced & ½ tbsp finely chopped red onion
- cracked black pepper to taste
- Salad
- 1 clove garlic & 8 large ripe black olive
- 2 boneless, skinless chicken breasts (4 o: each)
- 4 cups torn lettuce
- 1 navel orange, peeled, sliced

Directions:

1. For the dressing, add vinegar, oil, celery garlic, onion, and pepper into a small bowl and whisk well. Cover the bowl : chill until you need to use it.

2. Meanwhile, preheat a grill or broiler. T the garlic clove and rub it all over the chicken breasts and place the chicken (the grill. Cook for 5 minutes. Flip side and cook the other side for 5 minutes until well cooked inside.

3. Place the chicken on your cutting boa Let it cool for 5–8 minutes before slici

4. To assemble, divide the lettuce onto tv plates.

5. Divide the olives, oranges, and chicker slices equally and place them over the lettuce.

6. Distribute the dressing equally and po it over the salad.

7. Serve right away.

Pasta Salad With Dill

Time: 23 minutes

Serving Size: 4

Prep Time: 8 minutes

Cook Time: 8-15 minutes

Nutritional Facts Per Serving (¾ cup):

Calories: 160

Fat: 8 g

Total Carbohydrate: 23 g

Protein: 4 g

Sodium: 11 mg

Ingredients:

Dressing

2 tbsp olive oil

1 tbsp rice or white wine vinegar

cracked black pepper to taste

1 tbsp lemon juice & 1 tsp dill weed

Salad

1 ½ cups uncooked whole-grain shell pasta

½ cup halved cherry tomatoes

¼ cup chopped green onions

4 asparagus spears, cut into ½-inch pieces

½ cup sliced green bell pepper

Directions:

1. For the dressing, whisk together all the dressing ingredients in a bowl. Cover and keep it away for now.

2. Cook pasta following the directions given on the package. Add asparagus for 3 minutes before draining the pasta.

3. Combine pasta, bell pepper, tomatoes, and onion in a bowl. Pour dressing over the salad. Toss well, cover the bowl, and chill for at least a couple of hours. Serve.

Mixed Bean Salad

Time: 5 minutes

Serving Size: 4

Prep Time: 5 minutes

Cook Time: none

Nutritional Facts Per Serving (¼ recipe):

Calories: 113

Fat: 1.5 g

Total Carbohydrate: 19 g

Protein: 6 g

Sodium: 138 mg

Ingredients:

- ½ can unsalted chickpeas (from a 15-oz can), drained
- ½ can unsalted kidney beans (from a 15-oz can), drained
- ½ can unsalted wax beans (from a 15-oz can), drained
- ½ can unsalted green beans (from a 15-oz can), drained
- ⅛ cup chopped onion
- ¼ cup cider vinegar
- 2 tbsp orange juice
- sugar substitute to taste (optional)

Directions:

1. Add all the beans into a bowl. Add onion and stir. Add orange juice, vinegar, and sugar substitutes and mix well. Let it rest

for about 30 minutes.

2. Toss well and serve.

White Bean and Veggie Salad

Time: 10 minutes

Serving Size: 2

Prep Time: 10 minutes

Cook Time: none

Nutritional Facts Per Serving (4 cups):

Calories: 360

Fat: 24.6 g

Total Carbohydrate: 29.7 g

Protein: 10.1 g

Sodium: 321 mg

Ingredients:

- 4 cups mixed salad greens
- ⅔ cup unsalted canned white beans
- 2 tbsp red wine vinegar
- ½ tsp kosher salt
- 1 ½ cups mixture of chopped cucumber and halved cherry tomatoes
- 1 avocado, peeled, pitted, diced
- 4 tsp extra-virgin olive oil
- freshly ground pepper to taste

Directions:

1. Add mixed salad greens, beans, cucumber, tomatoes, and avocado into a bowl and toss well. Pour oil and vinegar over the salad and add salt and pepper.

2. Mix well and serve.

Peanut Dipping Sauce

Time: 5 minutes

Serving Size: 3

Prep Time: 5 minutes

Cook Time: none

Nutritional Facts Per Serving (⅓ recipe):

Calories: 55

Fat: 2.8 g

Total Carbohydrate: 4.8 g

Protein: 3 g

Sodium: 253 mg

Ingredients:

2 tbsp reduced-fat peanut butter

½ clove garlic, minced & ½ tsp sesame oil & ½ tbsp light soy sauce

½ tsp sugar

2 tbsp nonfat plain Greek yogurt

½ tsp minced fresh ginger & ½ tbsp apple cider vinegar

½ tbsp lime juice

⅛ tsp red pepper flakes (optional)

Directions:

Add peanut butter, garlic, sesame oil, soy sauce, sugar, yogurt, ginger, vinegar, lime juice, and red pepper flakes into a bowl and mix well.

Cover and set aside for a while for the flavors to meld. Add some water to get the desired consistency if the sauce is thick.

Tzatziki Sauce

Time: 10 minutes

Serving Size: 26

Prep Time: 10 minutes

Cook Time: none

Nutritional Facts Per Serving (2 tbsp):

Calories: 28

Fat: 0 g

Total Carbohydrate: 3 g

Protein: 4 g

Sodium: 41 mg

Ingredients:

- 4 large cucumbers, peeled, halved lengthwise, deseeded, grated, drained
- 9 tsp finely chopped fresh dill
- salt to taste
- 32 oz of fat-free plain Greek yogurt
- 1 tsp chopped garlic
- pepper to taste

Directions:

1. Combine yogurt, garlic, pepper, salt, and dill in a bowl. Cover and keep it in the refrigerator until use.

Savory Vegetable Dip

Time: 5 minutes

Serving Size: 4

Prep Time: 5 minutes

Cook Time: none

Nutritional Facts Per Serving (¼ cup without serving options):

Calories: 57

Fat: 1.5 g

Total Carbohydrate: 7 g

Protein: 4 g

Sodium: 222 mg

Ingredients:

- 2 small garlic cloves, peeled
- ½ cup fat-free cottage cheese
- 3 tbsp fat-free mayonnaise
- 6 tbsp chopped oil-packed, sun-dried tomatoes, drained and dried by patting with paper towels
- 3 tbsp plain fat-free yogurt

Directions:

1. Blend garlic, cottage cheese, mayonnaise, sun-dried tomatoes, and yogurt until smooth.
2. Serve with vegetable sticks or crackers, etc.

House Ranch Dressing

Time: 5 minutes

Serving Size: 10

Prep Time: 5 minutes

Cook Time: none

Nutritional Facts Per Serving (2 tbsp):

Calories: 30

Fat: 1 g

Total Carbohydrate: 2 g

Protein: 2 g

Sodium: 110 mg

Ingredients:

- 1 cup plain fat-free Greek yogurt
- 1 tbsp lemon juice
- ¾ tsp onion powder
- ¼ tsp kosher salt
- ¼ cup low-fat mayonnaise
- ½ tbsp dried dill weed
- ¾ tsp garlic powder
- ⅛ tsp pepper

Directions:

1. Blend yogurt, lemon juice, salt, herb an spices, and mayonnaise until smooth. P into an airtight container and refrigera until use. It can last for two weeks.

Pepper Sauce

Time: 1 hour 30 minutes

Serving Size: 5

Prep Time: 60 minutes

Cook Time: 30 minutes

Nutritional Facts Per Serving (about tbsp):

Calories: 64

Fat: 6 g

Total Carbohydrate: 2 g

Protein: 0.5 g

Sodium: 3 mg

Ingredients:

- ½ dried ancho chili pepper
- ½ dried New Mexico chili pepper
- ½ dried chipotle chili pepper
- ½ cup white wine vinegar
- 2 tbsp olive oil
- ¼ cup water
- ½ red fresh Fresno or jalapeño chili pepper

Directions:

1. Wear gloves while handling the chilies. Place dried chilies in a bowl. Drizzle vinegar and water over the chilies and let them soak for 1 hour.

2. Transfer into a saucepan along with Fresno chili and place it over low heat. Let it boil gently for about 20–25 minutes. Turn off the heat and allow it to cool for a few minutes.

3. Transfer the chilies to the small blender jar and blend until smooth. Pour oil in a thin drizzle through the feeder tube (with the machine running). Blend until well combined.

4. Transfer the sauce to an airtight container and refrigerate until use. It can last for about 12–15 days.

Peanut Butter Hummus

Time: 5 minutes

Serving Size: 8

Prep Time: 5 minutes

Cook Time: none

Nutritional Facts Per Serving (2 tbsp):

Calories: 135

Fat: 4 g

Total Carbohydrate: 19 g

Protein: 7 g

Sodium: 47 mg

Ingredients:

- 1 cup unsalted cooked or canned chickpeas
- ¼ cup powdered peanut butter
- 1 tbsp brown sugar
- ½ cup water
- 2 tbsp natural peanut butter
- ½ tsp vanilla extract

Directions:

1. Blend chickpeas, peanut butter powder, brown sugar, water, peanut butter, and vanilla until smooth.

2. Transfer into an airtight container and chill until use. It can last for a week.

Acorn Squash With Apples

Time: 10 minutes

Serving Size: 4

Prep Time: 5 minutes

Cook Time: 5 minutes

Nutritional Facts Per Serving (½ squash and ½ apple):

Calories: 204

Fat: 4 g

Total Carbohydrate: 40 g

Protein: 2 g

Sodium: 46 mg

Ingredients:

- 2 Granny Smith apples, peeled, cored, cut into slices
- 2 small acorn squashes (6 inches in diameter each)
- 4 tbsp brown sugar
- 4 tsp trans fat-free margarine

Directions:

1. Place apples in a bowl. Sprinkle brown sugar and mix well. Prick the squashes a few times with a sharp knife at several places. Cook the squashes in the microwave for 5 minutes or until tender. Turn the squashes over after about 3–4 minutes of cooking.

2. Once tender, bring it onto your cutting board. When it cools slightly, cut them into two halves. Remove the seeds from the squash halves. Place apple slices in the squash cavity and place the squash back in the microwave. Cook for a couple of minutes.

3. To serve, place a teaspoon of margarine on the apples in each squash and serve.

Creamed Swiss Chard

Time: 17 minutes

Serving Size: 4

Prep Time: 5 minutes

Cook Time: 10–12 minutes

Nutritional Facts Per Serving (about 1 ½ cups):

Calories: 101

Fat: 5 g

Total Carbohydrate: 8 g

Protein: 5 g

Sodium: 297 mg

Ingredients:

- 1 tbsp olive oil
- 2 small garlic cloves, finely chopped
- 1 lb Swiss chard, washed, stemmed, cut into ½-inch wide strips crosswise
- freshly ground pepper to taste
- 2 tsp all-purpose flour
- ⅔ cup low-fat plain soy milk
- ⅛ tsp salt
- 2 tsp grated Parmesan cheese

Directions:

1. Pour oil into a skillet and let it heat ove medium heat. When the oil is hot, add flour and whisk well. Add garlic and sau until you get a pleasant aroma.

2. Add soy milk. Keep whisking until thic

3. Add Swiss chard and mix well. Cover with a lid and let it cook until it wilts.

4. Turn off the heat and sprinkle salt and pepper and stir. Garnish with Parmesan cheese and serve.

Brown Rice Pilaf

Time: 38 minutes

Serving Size: 3

Prep Time: 5–8 minutes

Cook Time: 30 minutes

Nutritional Facts Per Serving (1 ¼ cups):

Calories: 172

Fat: 4 g

Total Carbohydrate: 29 g

Protein: 5 g

Sodium: 139 mg

Ingredients:

½ tbsp olive oil

1 ½ cups water

¼ cup chopped onion

a pinch of ground nutmeg

1 tbsp finely grated Swiss cheese

½ cup brown rice

½ tsp low-sodium, chicken-flavored bouillon granules

4 oz fresh mushrooms, thinly sliced

4 oz asparagus tips, cut into 1-inch pieces

¼ cup chopped fresh parsley

Directions:

Pour oil into a saucepan and let it heat over medium heat. When the oil is hot, mix the rice into the oil and cook until the rice is light brown. Add onion, water, nutmeg, mushrooms, and bouillon granules and stir.

When it starts boiling, turn down the heat and cook covered until tender. If the rice is uncooked and there is no water in the saucepan, add more water and cook until tender.

3. Stir in asparagus tips and keep the saucepan covered for about 4–5 minutes. Add cheese and stir. Sprinkle parsley on top and serve.

Braised Kale With Cherry Tomatoes

Time: 20 minutes

Serving Size: 3

Prep Time: 10 minutes

Cook Time: 10 minutes

Nutritional Facts Per Serving (1 ½ cups):

Calories: 70

Fat: 2 g

Total Carbohydrate: 9 g

Protein: 4 g

Sodium: 133 mg

Ingredients:

- 1 tsp extra-virgin olive oil
- ½ lb kale, tough stems removed, leaves chopped into small pieces
- ½ cup halved cherry tomatoes
- ⅛ tsp salt
- 2 garlic cloves, thinly sliced
- ¼ cup low-sodium vegetable stock or broth
- ½ tbsp lemon juice
- a pinch of freshly ground pepper or to taste

Directions:

1. Pour oil into a pan and place the pan over medium heat. When the oil is hot, add garlic and constantly stir for about a minute or until it turns light golden brown. Add kale and vegetable stock. Cook covered on medium-low heat until the kale has turned limp and the mixture is dry.

2. Add tomatoes and stir. Cook without covering for 5–6 minutes or until the kale is cooked. Turn off the heat.

3. Add lemon juice, salt, and pepper and mix well. Serve.

Cheesy Baked Zucchini

Time: 45 minutes

Serving Size: 4

Prep Time: 5 minutes

Cook Time: 35–40 minutes

Nutritional Facts Per Serving (1 zucchini half):

Calories: 52

Fat: 4 g

Total Carbohydrate: 4 g

Protein: 3 g

Sodium: 85 mg

Ingredients:

- 2 medium zucchinis (6 inches in length), trimmed, halved lengthwise
- ¼ tsp garlic powder
- 2 tsp olive oil
- 4 tbsp Parmesan cheese, grated
- ½ tsp onion powder

Directions:

1. Preheat the oven to 375 °F.

2. Take one zucchini half, and with a knife, slice crosswise at every ½ inch but not totally. It should be attached at the bottom (skin and a little zucchini flesh should be intact). Do this with the remaining zucchini halves.

3. Take four sheets of aluminum foil and place a zucchini half on each foil. Brush with oil generously and sprinkle garlic powder and onion powder over the zucchini halves. Wrap each foil to completely enclose the zucchini.

4. Place the foil packets on a baking sheet. And pop it into the oven for about 30 minutes or until fork tender. Take out the foil packet and set the oven to broil mode.

5. Open the foil. Sprinkle cheese over the zucchini. Lift the foil and place it back the oven.

6. Broil for a couple of minutes until the cheese is slightly brown.

7. Serve.

Honey Sage Carrots

Time: 13 minutes

Serving Size: 2

Prep Time: 5 minutes

Cook Time: 5–8 minutes

Nutritional Facts Per Serving (½ cup

Calories: 74

Fat: 2 g

Total Carbohydrate: 15 g

Protein: 1 g

Sodium: 112 mg

Ingredients:

- 1 cup sliced carrots
- 1 tbsp honey
- ⅛ tsp pepper
- 1 tsp butter
- ½ tbsp chopped fresh sage
- a pinch of salt

Directions:

1. Drop carrots in a pot of boiling water and let it cook for a few minutes until tender, and you can pierce them with a fork. Drain the carrots in a colander and keep them aside.

2. Add butter to a pan and let it melt over medium heat. Add carrots, pepper, sage, and honey when the butter melts and mix well. Cook for a couple of minutes and add a pinch of salt. Stir often.

3. Turn off the heat and serve.

Glazed Radishes

Time: 25 minutes

Serving Size: 2

Prep Time: 5 minutes

Cook Time: 20 minutes

Nutritional Facts Per Serving (½ recipe):

Calories: 150

: 12 g

Total Carbohydrate: 10 g

Protein: 2 g

Sodium: 295 mg

Ingredients:

- 1 tbsp olive oil, divided
- 1 tbsp unsalted butter at room temperature
- sesame seeds to garnish
- ¾ lb small–medium radishes, trimmed, halved
- ½ cup thinly sliced radish greens
- 1 tbsp white miso

Directions:

1. Preheat the oven to 450 °F. Prepare a baking sheet by greasing it with ½ tbsp of oil. Place radishes on the baking sheet with the skin side facing up. Trickle the remaining oil over the radishes.

2. Place the baking sheet in the oven and set the timer for 15 minutes until the radishes are cooked and the underside is golden brown.

3. Place miso and butter in a bowl and stir. Add radishes and toss well. Add radish greens and stir.

4. Garnish with sesame seeds and serve.

Chapter 7: Vegetable Plates

Pasta Primavera

Time: 25 minutes

Serving Size: 3

Prep Time: 10 minutes

Cook Time: 15 minutes

Nutritional Facts Per Serving (1 cup of pasta with 1 cup of vegetables):

Calories: 347

Fat: 7 g

Total Carbohydrate: 54 g

Protein: 17 g

Sodium: 223 mg

Ingredients:

- 1 cup broccoli florets
- ½ cup sliced zucchini or yellow squash
- ½ tbsp extra-virgin olive oil
- 1 garlic clove, minced & ½ cup evaporated fat-free milk
- 6 oz of whole wheat pasta or angel hair pasta spaghetti
- 1 cup sliced bell pepper of any color
- ¼ cup chopped onion
- ½ tsp butter & 6 tbsp freshly grated Parmesan cheese
- 3 tbsp finely chopped parsley

Directions:

1. Pour an inch of water into a pot. Place a steamer basket in the pot. Place broccoli, zucchini, mushrooms, and peppers in the steamer basket and cover the pot. Steam for about 6–8 minutes or until th vegetables are crisp and tender. Take out the steamer basket and remove the pot from the heat.

2. Add butter into a saucepan and place it over medium heat. Add evaporated milk and Parmesan cheese and keep stirring until very hot. Turn off the heat and kee it covered.

3. Meanwhile, cook pasta following the directions given on the package.

4. Distribute the pasta into two plates. Plac steamed vegetables over the pasta. Divid the sauce equally and pour it over the pasta and vegetables.

5. Serve.

Polenta With Fresh Vegetables

Time: 50 minutes

Serving Size: 2

Prep Time: 10 minutes

Cook Time: 40 minutes

Nutritional Facts Per Serving (1 cup polenta with 1 cup of vegetables):

Calories: 178

Fat: 1 g

Total Carbohydrate: 34 g

Protein: 6 g

Sodium: 55 mg

Ingredients:

½ cup coarsely ground cornmeal (polenta)

½ tsp chopped garlic

½ cup sliced onions

½ cup sliced zucchini

chopped fresh herbs of your choice to garnish

2 cups water

½ cup sliced fresh mushrooms

½ cup broccoli florets

1 tbsp grated Parmesan cheese

Directions:

Preheat the oven to 350 °F. Grease an ovenproof dish with cooking spray. Add polenta, garlic, and water into the dish and mix well.

Place the baking dish in the oven and bake for about 40 minutes or until the polenta comes off from the sides of the baking dish. The polenta should not be dry so bake accordingly.

Meanwhile, place a nonstick pan over medium heat. Spray some cooking spray into the pan. When the pan is hot, add onion and mushrooms and mix well. Stir on and off until the veggies are cooked.

Pour an inch of water into a pot. Place a steamer basket in the pot. Place broccoli and zucchini in the steamer basket and cover the pot. Steam for about 10 minutes or until the vegetables are crisp and tender.

Place the polenta on individual serving plates. Place cooked vegetables on top. Garnish with Parmesan and fresh herbs and serve.

Quinoa Risotto With Arugula and Parmesan

Time: 23 minutes

Serving Size: 3

Prep Time: 5–8 minutes

Cook Time: 15 minutes

Nutritional Facts Per Serving (1 cup):

Calories: 161

Fat: 5 g

Total Carbohydrate: 22 g

Protein: 6 g

Sodium: 211 mg

Ingredients:

- ½ tbsp olive oil
- 1 small clove of garlic, minced
- 1 cup plus 2 tbsp low-sodium vegetable stock or broth
- ½ small carrot, finely shredded
- 2 tbsp Parmesan cheese, grated
- freshly ground pepper to taste
- ⅛ tsp salt or to taste
- ¼ cup finely chopped onion
- ½ cup quinoa, rinsed
- 1 cup chopped arugula
- ¼ cup sliced shiitake mushrooms

Directions:

1. Pour oil into a saucepan and let it heat over medium heat. When the oil is hot, add onion and cook until the onion is soft. Stir in the garlic and quinoa and sauté for a minute.

2. Next goes the stock. Add it to the saucepan and give it a good stir. When

it starts boiling, turn down the heat and simmer until the quinoa is nearly tender. Add carrot, arugula, and mushroom and stir. Cook until all the stock has been absorbed.

3. Add cheese, salt, and pepper. Mix well and serve.

Vegetable Calzone

Time: 35 minutes

Serving Size: 2

Prep Time: 15 minutes

Cook Time: 15–20 minutes

Nutritional Facts Per Serving (1 calzone with 2 ½ tbsp of pizza sauce):

Calories: 264

Fat: 8 g

Total Carbohydrate: 36 g

Protein: 12 g

Sodium: 590 mg

Ingredients:

- 1 ½ stalks of asparagus, cut into 1-inch pieces
- ¼ cup chopped broccoli
- 1 tbsp minced garlic
- 4 oz frozen whole wheat bread dough, thawed
- ¼ cup shredded part-skim mozzarella cheese
- ¼ cup chopped spinach
- ¼ cup sliced mushrooms
- 1 tsp olive oil, divided
- ½ medium tomato, sliced
- ⅓ cup pizza sauce

Directions:

1. Preheat the oven to 400 °F. Spray some cooking spray on a baking sheet.

2. Combine all the vegetables and garlic in a nonstick pan. Add ½ tsp of oil and stir well. Cook the vegetables over medium-high heat until the vegetables are tender. Stir on and off. Turn off the heat and let it cool.

3. Meanwhile, dust your countertop with some flour. Cut the bread dough into two halves. Shape into rounds.

4. Now roll the dough thinly, with a rolling pin, into an oval shape. Do this with both dough halves.

5. Place half the vegetable mixture on one half of each rolled dough, leaving about ½-inch border all over. Divide the tomato and cheese equally and place them over the vegetable mixture. Moisten the edges of the rolled dough along the border. Fold the other half of the dough over the filling so it falls over the edges. Press the edges to seal well. Crimp the edges with fork and place it on the baking sheet.

6. Place the baking sheet in the oven and set the timer for 10–12 minutes or until golden brown.

7. Serve calzone with warm pizza sauce.

Eggplant Parmesan

Time: 42 minutes

Serving Size: 3

Prep Time: 10–12 minutes

Cook Time: 30 minutes

Nutritional Facts Per Serving (1 ½ cups):

Calories: 241

Fat: 9 g

Total Carbohydrate: 28 g

Protein: 14 g

Sodium: 553 mg

Ingredients:

1 large egg

½ cup panko breadcrumbs & ½ tsp Italian seasoning

¼ tsp salt

½ jar (from a 24-oz jar) of unsalted tomato sauce

1 garlic clove, grated

½ cup shredded part-skim mozzarella cheese, divided

1 tbsp water & 6 tbsp grated Parmesan cheese, divided

1 lb eggplants, cut into ¼-inch thick slices crosswise

¼ tsp pepper

⅛ cup torn fresh basil leaves plus extra to garnish

¼ tsp crushed red pepper

Directions:

Preheat the oven to 400 °F. Spray some cooking spray on a baking sheet and a baking dish.

2. Beat egg in a bowl, adding water. Place breadcrumbs, Italian seasoning, and 2 tbsp of Parmesan cheese in a shallow bowl and mix well.

3. Working with one eggplant slice at a time, dunk it in egg. Shake off excess egg and dredge the eggplant slice in breadcrumbs. Press while dredging. Place the eggplant slices on the baking sheet.

4. Spray the eggplant slices with cooking spray. Flip the sides and spray the other side as well. Place the baking sheet in the oven and set the timer for 30 minutes or until light brown. Sprinkle salt and pepper over the eggplant slices.

5. Add tomato sauce, garlic, basil, and red pepper into a bowl and stir. Spread a thin layer of this sauce on the bottom of the prepared baking sheet.

6. Place half the eggplant slices in the baking dish. Spread ½ cup of sauce mixture over the eggplant slices. Scatter 2 tbsp of Parmesan and 4 tbsp of mozzarella over the eggplant slices.

7. Place the remaining eggplant slices in the dish. Spread all the sauce that is remaining over the eggplant slices. Sprinkle the remaining cheese on top and place it in the oven.

8. Set the timer for 20–30 minutes or until golden brown on top. Let the baking dish rest on your countertop for 5 minutes. Serve.

Chickpea Pasta With Spinach

Time: 32 minutes

Serving Size: 3

Prep Time: 5–7 minutes

Cook Time: 20–25 minutes

Nutritional Facts Per Serving (2 ½ cups):

Calories: 283

Fat: 7 g

Total Carbohydrate: 44 g

Protein: 11 g

Sodium: 130 mg

Ingredients:

- 1 ½ cups dry bow tie pasta
- 2 garlic cloves, crushed
- ¼ cup unsalted chicken broth
- 2 cups chopped fresh spinach
- cracked black pepper to taste
- 1 tbsp olive oil
- ¼ can (from a 19-oz can) of chickpeas, rinsed, drained
- ¼ cup golden raisins
- 1 tbsp grated Parmesan cheese

Directions:

1. Follow the directions given on the package of the pasta and cook it accordingly.
2. Pour oil into a skillet and let it heat over medium heat. When the oil is hot, add garlic and cook for a few seconds without browning.
3. Stir in the chickpeas and broth. Cook for about a minute.
4. Stir in the spinach and raisins and cook until the spinach turns limp. Make sure you do not overcook the spinach.
5. Add pasta, cheese, and pepper and toss well. Serve right away.

Chapter 8: Vegan Plate Recipes

Black Bean and Sweet Potato Rice Bowls

Time: 28 minutes

Serving Size: 2

Prep Time: 5–8 minutes

Cook Time: 20 minutes

Nutritional Facts Per Serving (2 cups):

Calories: 435

Fat: 11 g

Total Carbohydrate: 74 g

Protein: 10 g

Sodium: 405 mg

Ingredients:

- 6 tbsp uncooked long-grain rice
- ¾ cup water
- ½ large sweet potato, peeled, diced
- 2 cups fresh kale, chopped
- 1 tbsp sweet chili sauce plus extra to serve
- ⅛ tsp garlic salt & 1 ½ tbsp olive oil, divided
- ½ medium red onion, finely chopped
- ½ can (from a 15-oz can) of black beans, rinsed, drained
- Lemon wedges to serve

Directions:

Add rice, salt, garlic, and water into a saucepan and place the saucepan over medium heat. When it starts boiling, turn down the heat and cover it with a lid. Simmer until the rice is cooked and no water is left in the saucepan. Turn off the heat and let it rest covered for 5 minutes. Add chili sauce and ½ tbsp of oil and stir lightly until well combined. Cover and set aside for now.

2. Pour a tablespoon of oil into a skillet and let it heat over medium-high heat. When the oil is hot, add sweet potato and stir well. Cook for about 7–8 minutes.

3. Stir in the onion and cook until you can pierce the sweet potato easily with a fork. Stir in the kale and cook for a few minutes until the kale wilts. Add beans and mix well. Let it heat thoroughly.

4. Add rice and mix well. Divide the rice into two plates. Place a lime wedge on each plate. Drizzle some chili sauce on top and serve.

Black Bean and Corn Quinoa

Time: 30 minutes

Serving Size: 2

Prep Time: 8–10 minutes

Cook Time: 20 minutes

Nutritional Facts Per Serving (1 ¼ cups):

Calories: 375

Fat: 10 g

Total Carbohydrate: 16 g

Protein: 13 g

Sodium: 60 mg

Ingredients:

- 1 tbsp canola oil
- ½ medium red bell pepper, finely chopped
- 1 tsp chili powder
- ⅛ tsp pepper
- ½ cup frozen corn
- ½ can (from a 15-oz can) of black beans, rinsed, drained
- ½ medium onion, finely chopped
- ½ celery rib, finely chopped
- ⅛ tsp salt & 1 cup vegetable stock
- ½ cup quinoa, rinsed
- 4 tbsp minced fresh cilantro, divided

Directions:

1. Pour oil into a skillet and let it heat over medium-high heat. When the oil is hot, add bell pepper, onion, celery, chili powder, and pepper and mix well. Cook for 5–6 minutes.

2. Add stock and stir. When it starts boiling, add corn and quinoa and stir. Turn down the heat and cover with a lid. Cook until there is no broth left in the pot.

3. Stir in cilantro and beans. Turn off the heat and let it sit covered for 5 minutes.

4. Fluff the grains with a fork. Garnish with some more cilantro and serve.

Southwestern Bowl

Time: 1 hour 12 minutes

Serving Size: 3

Prep Time: 10–12 minutes

Cook Time: 45–60 minutes

Nutritional Facts Per Serving (2 cups)

Calories: 376

Fat: 4 g

Total Carbohydrate: 68 g

Protein: 18 g

Sodium: 67 mg

Ingredients:

- 1 tsp canola oil
- 1 cup chopped green bell pepper
- 1 garlic clove, minced
- ½ cup tomato, chopped
- ½ cup red onion, chopped
- 1 small chili pepper, chopped
- ½ cup sweet potato cubes
- 2 cups kale, hard ribs and stems discarded, chopped
- a handful of fresh cilantro, chopped
- ¼ cup green lentils
- ½ cup brown rice
- ¼ cup red lentils
- ½ tbsp ground cumin
- 1 cup vegetable stock, unsalted
- ½ tbsp freshly ground pepper
- 1 cup water
- ½ tbsp red wine vinegar
- ½ cup cooked black beans
- lime wedges to serve

Directions:

1. Pour oil into a skillet and let it heat over medium-high heat. When the oil is hot, add onion, garlic, pepper, sweet potato, and tomatoes and cook until the onions are translucent.

2. Add rice, green lentils, red lentils, all the spices, stock, vinegar, and water and stir. When it starts boiling, turn down the heat and cover it with a lid. Simmer until soft but not mushy. It can take a long time to cook. If you have an instant pot or pressure cooker, you can cook this recipe in it. It will be much quicker.

3. Add kale, black beans, and cilantro and mix well. Serve with lime wedges.

Rice Noodles With Spring Vegetables

Time: 23 minutes

Serving Size: 3

Prep Time: 6–8 minutes

Cook Time: 15 minutes

Nutritional Facts Per Serving (1 ½ cups):

Calories: 205

Fat: 5 g

Total Carbohydrate: 37 g

Protein: 3 g

Sodium: 215 mg

Ingredients:

- ½ tbsp peanut oil
- ½ tbsp fresh ginger, grated
- 1 tbsp low-sodium soy sauce
- ½ cup fresh bean sprouts
- ½ cup fresh spinach, chopped
- crushed red chili flakes to serve
- 4 oz rice noodles
- ½ tbsp sesame oil
- 1 garlic clove, finely chopped
- ½ cup small broccoli florets
- 4 cherry tomatoes, halved
- 1 scallion, chopped

Directions:

1. Follow the directions given on the package of the noodles and cook it accordingly.

2. Pour sesame and peanut oil into a skillet or wok and let it heat over medium heat. Stir the ginger and garlic into the oil and cook for a few seconds, stirring often. Add soy sauce and broccoli and mix well. Cook for a couple of minutes.

3. Add noodles, scallion, tomatoes, bean sprouts, and spinach and toss well. Heat thoroughly.

4. Garnish with crushed red chili flakes and serve.

Yellow Lentils With Spinach and Ginger

Time: 53 minutes (soaking time included)

Serving Size: 2

Prep Time: 5 minutes plus 30 minutes soaking time (optional)

Cook Time: 15–18 minutes

Nutritional Facts Per Serving (¾ cup):

Calories: 263

Fat: 7 g

Total Carbohydrate: 36 g

Protein: 14 g

Sodium: 348 mg

Ingredients:

- ½ tbsp olive oil
- ½ tsp ground ginger
- ¼ tsp turmeric powder
- ¼ tsp curry powder
- ½ minced shallot
- ½ cup yellow lentils, picked, rinsed, drained, and soaked in water for 30 minutes if possible
- ¼ cup light coconut milk
- ¼ tsp salt & ¾ cup unsalted vegetable stock
- 1 cup chopped baby spinach leaves
- ½ tbsp chopped fresh cilantro
- ½ tsp white or black sesame seeds, toasted

Directions:

1. Pour oil into a saucepan and place it over medium heat. When the oil is hot, add shallot and spices and mix well. Cook for a few seconds, making sure not to burn the spices.

2. Stir in lentils, coconut milk, and stock. When the mixture starts boiling, turn down the heat and cover the saucepan partially with a lid. Cook until the lentils are soft yet firm. If there is not much liquid in the saucepan, add some water.

3. Add spinach and mix well. Cover the pot

and cook for a couple of minutes until the spinach wilts. Add salt and mix well. Sprinkle cilantro and sesame seeds on to and serve.

Sesame-Crusted Tofu

Time: 25 minutes

Serving Size: 2

Prep Time: 15 minutes

Cook Time: 10 minutes

Nutritional Facts Per Serving (3 slices of tofu):

Calories: 258

Fat: 14 g

Total Carbohydrate: 14 g

Protein: 19 g

Sodium: 124 mg

Ingredients:

- ½ lb firm tofu, drained, cut into six equ slices
- 1 egg white
- 1 ½ tbsp plain dried breadcrumbs
- ½ tbsp black sesame seeds
- 1 tbsp white sesame seeds
- 6 green onions, trimmed, halved lengthwise and crosswise
- ⅛ cup fat-free milk
- ⅛ tsp freshly ground pepper
- ¼ tsp sesame oil or canola oil
- ¾ tsp sriracha sauce

rections:

.Place a paper towel on a plate. Place a slice of tofu over it. Place another paper towel over the tofu slice. Repeat this stacking of tofu and paper towels. Let it sit for 10 minutes. Now take off the paper napkins.

Heat a nonstick pan over medium heat. Add tofu slices in a single layer and cook until the underside is slightly brown. Flip sides and cook the other side until light brown. Turn off the heat. Remove the tofu from the pan and place it on a plate to cool.

Add egg white, milk, and pepper into a bowl and whisk well. Place breadcrumbs and sesame seeds in a shallow bowl and stir well.

Working with one tofu slice at a time, dunk the tofu slice in the egg mixture. Shake off the excess egg and roll in the sesame seed mixture.

Place the pan over medium heat. Add oil and let it heat. When the oil is hot, place the tofu slices in the pan. Cook until the underside is light brown. Flip the sides and cook the other side as well. Remove the tofu from the pan and place it on a plate.

Next, cook the green onion in the pan until it wilts. Divide the green onions equally and place them into two plates. Place three tofu slices on each plate over the green onion. Drizzle sriracha sauce on top and serve.

Chapter 9: Bread Recipes

Whole Wheat Bread

Time: 40 minutes

Serving Size: 2 loaves (24 slices each)

Prep Time: 10 minutes

Cook Time: 30 minutes

Nutritional Facts Per Serving (1 slice):

Calories: 85

Fat: 1 g

Total Carbohydrate: 15 g

Protein: 4 g

Sodium: 170 mg

Ingredients:

- 3 cups all-purpose flour plus extra for dusting and kneading
- 4 cups whole wheat flour
- 1 cup wheat germ
- ½ tsp salt
- 2 eggs, lightly beaten
- 4 cups low-fat buttermilk
- 4 tsp baking soda

Directions:

1. Preheat the oven to 400 °F.
2. Add all-purpose flour, whole wheat flour, baking soda, wheat germ, and salt into a mixing bowl and mix well.
3. Whisk in the eggs and buttermilk. You will get sticky dough; don't worry. Dust your countertop with a good amount of flour. Place the dough on the dusted area. Dust your hands with flour as well. Knead the dough for about 30–40 seconds.
4. Divide the dough into two equal portions and shape it into balls.
5. Take a large baking sheet and place the dough balls on either side of the baking sheet. Pat the dough lightly to give it a round shape of about 7 inches in diameter. Make sure there is sufficient space between the dough. Sprinkle some flour over the dough.
6. With your finger pushed in the dough about ½-inch deep, make an X mark on top of each dough.
7. Place the baking sheet in the oven and set the timer for 25–30 minutes or until baked. You should hear a hollow sound when you tap the bread on the bottom. Place the bread on a wire rack for cooling.
8. Cut each bread into 24 slices and store an airtight container.

Herb–Parmesan Bread

Time: 58 minutes

Serving Size: 2 loaves (16 slices each)

Prep Time: 8 minutes

Cook Time: 50 minutes

Nutritional Facts Per Serving (1 slice)

Calories: 136

Fat: 6 g

Total Carbohydrate: 16 g

rotein: 4 g

odium: 230 mg

agredients:

- 4 cups white whole wheat flour
- 4 tsp baking powder
- 1 cup ground flaxseeds or flaxseed meal
- ½ tsp salt & 1 tsp baking soda
- 2 eggs, lightly beaten
- ½ cup vegetable oil & 3 cups buttermilk
- 1 cup grated Parmesan cheese plus ½ cup to top
- 2 tbsp chopped fresh thyme
- ½ cup chopped fresh parsley
- 4–5 garlic cloves, minced
- ½ tsp garlic powder

rections:

.Preheat the oven to 350 °F. Grease two loaf pans of 9 by 5 inches each with cooking spray and set aside.

.Add all the dry ingredients into a bowl (i.e., flour, baking powder, garlic powder, minced garlic, Parmesan, flaxseeds, thyme, parsley, salt, and baking soda) and mix well. You can add any other herbs instead of these herbs if desired.

Whisk together buttermilk, oil, and eggs in a bowl. Pour into the bowl of dry ingredients and mix until well combined.

Divide the batter into the prepared loaf pans. Sprinkle ¼ cup Parmesan cheese on each loaf. Bake in batches if required.

Place the loaf pans in the oven and set the timer for about 40–50 minutes or until a toothpick inserted in the center of the bread has no batter stuck on it when you

pull it out. Let it cool until it is warm.

6.Remove the loaves from the pan, cut each loaf into 16 equal slices, and serve. Store the bread slices in an airtight container.

Whole-Grain Banana Bread (Vegan)

Time: 50 minutes

Serving Size: 1 loaf (7 slices)

Prep Time: 10 minutes

Cook Time: 40 minutes

Nutritional Facts Per Serving (1 slice):

Calories: 150

Fat: 3 g

Total Carbohydrate: 30 g

Protein: 4 g

Sodium: 150 mg

Ingredients:

- ¼ cup brown rice flour
- ¼ cup tapioca flour
- ¼ cup quinoa flour
- ¼ cup amaranth flour
- ¼ cup millet flour
- ¼ tsp baking powder & ½ tsp baking soda
- a pinch of salt
- 1 tbsp grape-seed oil
- 1 cup mashed banana
- 6 tbsp egg substitute or egg whites
- ¼ cup raw sugar

Directions:

1. Preheat the oven to 350 °F. Grease a small loaf pan with cooking spray. Sprinkle a little of any of the flour and keep it aside.
2. Add flour, baking powder, soda, and salt into a bowl.
3. Whisk together egg, sugar, oil, and banana in a bowl. Add the egg mixture into the bowl of the flour mixture and mix until well combined. Scoop the batter into the prepared loaf pan.
4. Place the loaf pan in the oven and set the timer for about 30–40 minutes or until a toothpick inserted in the center comes out clean.
5. Cut into seven equal slices and serve. You can store the bread slices in an airtight container.

Chocolate Chip Bread

Time: 58 minutes

Serving Size: 2 loaves (16 slices each)

Prep Time: 8 minutes

Cook Time: 50 minutes

Nutritional Facts Per Serving (1 slice):

Calories: 164

Fat: 7 g

Total Carbohydrate: 25 g

Protein: 4 g

Sodium: 166 mg

Ingredients:

- 3 ⅓ cups white whole wheat flour
- 4 tsp baking powder
- ⅔ cup cocoa powder
- 1 cup ground flaxseeds or flaxseed meal
- ½ tsp salt
- 1 tsp baking soda & 2 eggs, lightly beaten
- 2 tsp vanilla extract
- ½ cup vegetable oil
- 3 cups buttermilk
- ¾ cup sugar
- 1 cup mini semisweet chocolate chips

Directions:

1. Preheat the oven to 350 °F. Grease two loaf pans of 9 by 5 inches each with cooking spray and set aside.
2. Add all the dry ingredients into a bowl (i.e., flour, baking powder, cocoa powder, flaxseeds, salt, and baking soda) and mix well.
3. Whisk together buttermilk, oil, vanilla, sugar, and eggs in a bowl. Pour into the bowl of dry ingredients and mix until well combined. Fold in the chocolate chips.
4. Divide the batter into the prepared loaf pans. Bake in batches if required.
5. Place the loaf pans in the oven and set timer for about 40–50 minutes or until a toothpick inserted in the center of the bread has no batter stuck on it when you pull it out. Let it cool until it is warm.
6. Remove the loaves from the pan, cut each loaf into 16 equal slices, and serve.

Whole Wheat Pretzels

Time: 50 minutes (rising time not included)

Serving Size: 2 loaves (14 slices each)

Prep Time: 20 minutes plus rising time

Cook Time: 30 minutes

Nutritional Facts Per Serving (1 slice):

Calories: 182

Fat: 2 g

Total Carbohydrate: 31 g

Protein: 10 g

Sodium: 108 mg

Ingredients:

2 packages of active dry yeast

1 tsp kosher salt

6 cups whole wheat flour

2 cups bread flour

1 cup wheat gluten

4 tbsp baking soda

4 tsp brown sugar

3 cups warm water

2 tbsp olive oil

2 egg whites or ½ cup egg substitute

2 tbsp sesame seeds, poppy seeds, flaxseeds, or sunflower seeds

To cook pretzels

¼ cup baking soda

8–10 cups water or as required

Directions:

Make the dough using your hands or in the food processor.

To make in the food processor, fit the dough hook attachment in the bowl, and you will have to make the dough in two batches.

3. Pour warm water into a bowl. Add yeast, salt, and sugar. Set aside for 5 minutes.

4. Combine bread flour, whole wheat flour, and wheat gluten in a bowl.

5. Place half the flour mixture in the food processor. Pour half the water mixture into the food processor and half the oil. Process until dough is formed.

6. Repeat the previous step once again. Spray two large bowls with cooking spray. Place a ball of dough in each bowl. Keep the bowl covered with cling wrap. Place the bowls in a warm area for a couple of hours until the dough rises to twice its original size.

7. Preheat the oven to 350 °F. Prepare two baking sheets by lining them with parchment paper.

8. With your fist, punch the dough balls. Divide each dough ball into 14 equal portions. Make balls of each portion.

9. Working with one ball of dough at a time, hold it in between your palms and roll it to make a long rope. Shape it into a pretzel.

10. Line two to three baking sheets with parchment paper. Place the pretzels on the baking sheet.

11. Add baking soda and 8–10 cups of water into a pot. Place the pot over high heat. When it comes to a rapid boil, bring it to a boil.

12. Drop the pretzels in the boiling water, one at a time, and remove after 30 seconds using a slotted spoon. Place the pretzels on the baking sheets.

13. Brush egg white or egg substitute over the pretzels. By using an egg substitute, you can make the pretzels vegan. Scatter the seeds on the pretzels.

14. Bake the pretzels in batches until the pretzels turn dark brown, for about 10–15 minutes.

Cinnamon Rolls

Time: 27 minutes (rising time not included)

Serving Size: 16

Prep Time: 10–12 minutes plus rising time

Cook Time: 15 minutes

Nutritional Facts Per Serving (1 cinnamon roll):

Calories: 130

Fat: 2 g

Total Carbohydrate: 25 g

Protein: 3 g

Sodium: 30 mg

Ingredients:

- ½ cup skim milk
- 3 tbsp sugar
- 6 tbsp brown sugar
- 1 package dry yeast
- 1 egg white
- 1 small egg
- 1 ¼ cups whole wheat flour
- 1 ½ cups all-purpose flour
- 1 tbsp ground cinnamon
- ¼ cup frozen unsweetened apple juice concentrate
- 2 tbsp canola oil
- ⅛ tsp salt
- 2 tbsp warm water
- ⅛ cup raisins

Directions:

1. Pour milk into a saucepan and heat un[til] very hot but not boiling. It should be less than the boiling point. Add white sugar, canola oil, and salt and mix well. Turn off the heat and let it cool until i[t] lukewarm.

2. Add yeast and warm water into a bowl and stir. Let it sit for about 5 minutes. [It] should be frothy by then.

3. Add egg and egg white into a bowl an[d] beat with an electric hand mixer until smooth. Stir in the yeast mixture using a wooden spoon. Add the flour mixtur[e] a cup at a time, and mix well each tim[e.] You should get a soft dough. You can also make the dough in a food process[or] or stand mixer with a dough hook attachment.

4. Dust your countertop with some flou[r] and place the dough on it. Knead for [a] few minutes until the dough is supple. Place the dough back in the bowl. Ke[ep] the bowl covered with cling wrap asid[e] in a warm place until it is about twice [the] original size.

5. Add raisins, cinnamon, and brown sug[ar] into a bowl and mix well. Grease a ba[king] dish of about 8–9 inches with cookin[g] spray.

6. Dust more flour on the countertop an[d] roll the dough with a rolling pin into a rectangle (16 by 8 inches). Spray the dough with some cooking spray. Spri[nkle]

the cinnamon sugar mixture all over the rolled dough.

7. Roll the dough into a log starting from the length of the rectangle. Cut into 16 equal slices and place them in the baking dish upright. Cover the dish loosely with cling wrap and keep it aside for about 1 ½ hours or until the rolls increase in size by almost twice.

8. Cook the apple juice concentrate in a saucepan until it is like syrup.

9. Preheat the oven to 350 °F. Brush the apple syrup over the rolls and put the baking dish into the oven. Set the timer for about 15 minutes or until the rolls are golden brown.

10. Take out the baking dish from the oven and let it cool. Serve warm.

Southwestern Cornmeal Muffins

Time: 47 minutes

Serving Size: 24

Prep Time: 5–7 minutes

Cook Time: 40 minutes

Nutritional Facts Per Serving (1 muffin):

Calories: 167

Fat: 5 g

Total Carbohydrate: 26 g

Protein: 4 g

Sodium: 138 mg

Ingredients:

- 2 ½ cups stone-ground cornmeal
- 2 cups all-purpose flour
- 4 tsp baking powder
- 1 cup egg substitute
- ½ cup vegetable oil
- 1 green bell pepper, finely chopped
- ½ cup sugar
- 2 cups fat-free milk
- 2 cups fresh or cream-style corn

Directions:

1. Preheat the oven to 350 °F. Prepare two muffin pans of 12 counts each by lining the cups with disposable paper liners or foil liners.

2. Add cornmeal, all-purpose flour, and baking powder into a bowl. Mix well.

3. Add egg substitute, oil, sugar, and milk into another bowl and mix well. Add bell pepper and corn and stir well. Pour the milk mixture into the flour mixture. Mix until just combined, without overmixing. If there are a few lumps in the batter, that is perfectly okay.

4. Pour batter into the muffin cups, filling up to two thirds. Place the muffin pans in the oven and set the timer for about 30–40 minutes or until a toothpick inserted in the center has no batter stuck on it when you take it out. The top should be light brown.

5. When done, place on a wire rack to cool completely. Then serve.

6. Place leftover muffins in an airtight container and refrigerate until use. It can last for five to six days in the refrigerator. Warm it slightly in the microwave and serve.

Raspberry Chocolate Scones (Vegan)

Time: 24 minutes

Serving Size: 24

Prep Time: 10–12 minutes

Cook Time: 12 minutes (per batch)

Nutritional Facts Per Serving (1 scone):

Calories: 149

Fat: 5 g

Total Carbohydrate: 22 g

Protein: 4 g

Sodium: 143 mg

Ingredients:

- 2 cups all-purpose flour
- 2 cups whole wheat pastry flour
- ½ tsp baking soda
- 2 tbsp baking powder
- ⅔ cup vegan butter
- ⅛ cup mini vegan chocolate chips
- 4 tbsp agave nectar or pure maple syrup
- ½ tsp ground cinnamon
- 1 cup fresh or frozen raspberries
- 2 ¼ cups nondairy yogurt
- 1 tsp raw sugar

Directions:

1. Preheat the oven to 350 °F. Grease two large baking sheets with cooking spray.

2. Add flour, baking soda and powder, and cinnamon into a bowl and stir. Add vegan butter and cut it into the mixture using a pastry cutter. You should get small crumbs.

3. Add nondairy yogurt and agave into a bowl and mix well. Pour it into the bowl of the flour mixture. Stir until just incorporated, making sure not to overm the dough.

4. Dust your countertop with a little flour. Turn the dough onto the floured area. Knead the dough a couple of times.

5. Divide the dough into balls. Roll each ball into a circle of about ½-inch thickness. Cut each dough into 12 equa wedges.

6. Place the wedges on the baking sheet, leaving a sufficient gap between them. Combine cinnamon and sugar in a bow and scatter over the scones. Bake in batches.

7. Place the baking sheet in the oven and set the timer for 10–12 minutes. Cool f a few minutes and serve. Store leftover scones in an airtight container.

8. If you do not want to make it vegan, yo can use regular butter, yogurt, and hone

Chapter 10: Fish and Shellfish Recipes

Halibut With Tomato Salsa

Time: 20 minutes

Serving Size: 2

Prep Time: 5 minutes

Cook Time: 15 minutes

Nutritional Facts Per Serving (½ recipe):

Calories: 140

Fat: 4 g

Total Carbohydrate: 4 g

Protein: 22 g

Sodium: 84 mg

Ingredients:

¾ cup diced tomatoes

½ tsp chopped fresh oregano

1 tsp extra-virgin olive oil

1 tbsp chopped fresh basil

½ tbsp minced garlic

2 halibut fillets, 4 oz each

Directions:

1. Preheat the oven to 350 °F. Grease a baking dish (about 8 inches) with cooking spray.

2. To make the salsa, add tomato, oil, herbs, and garlic into a bowl and mix well.

3. Place the halibut in the baking dish. Spread the salsa over the fish and place the baking dish in the oven.

4. Set the timer for 10–15 minutes or until the fish is cooked. When you pierce the fish with a fork, it should flake easily.

5. Serve hot.

Salmon and Asparagus Farro Bowl

Time: 38 minutes

Serving Size: 2

Prep Time: 8 minutes

Cook Time: 30 minutes

Nutritional Facts Per Serving (1 ½ cups salmon mixture with ½ cup farro):

Calories: 407

Fat: 11 g

Total Carbohydrate: 40 g

Protein: 37 g

Sodium: 432 mg

Ingredients:

- 6 tbsp farro
- 1 ½ cups water
- ½ tbsp extra-virgin olive oil
- ½ bunch of asparagus, trimmed, cut into 1-inch pieces
- 1 cup low-sodium chicken broth
- 10 oz wild Alaskan salmon fillet, skinless, cut into 1-inch pieces
- ⅛ tsp pepper
- ½ tbsp extra-virgin olive oil

- 1 ½ tbsp white miso
- 1 cup halved, thinly sliced leeks (white and light green parts only)
- 1 ½ tbsp thinly sliced fresh basil

Directions:

1. Add farro and water into a saucepan and bring the mixture to boil over high heat. Bring down the heat and cook until al dente. It should be chewy as well. Drain and set aside.
2. Pour oil into a saucepan and place it over medium heat after about 15 minutes of placing the farro saucepan over heat.
3. When the oil is hot, add leeks and stir. Cook until the leeks are slightly soft. Stir in the garlic and asparagus and cook for a few minutes. When the asparagus turns bright green, stir in miso and broth. Turn up the heat to high.
4. When it starts boiling, turn down the heat to medium heat. Add salmon and mix gently. Cook for 3 minutes. Turn off the heat. Add basil and pepper.
5. To assemble, serve ½ cup farro in each deep bowl. Ladle 1 ½ cups of the asparagus mixture into each bowl and serve.

Green Curry Salmon With Green Beans

Time: 30 minutes

Serving Size: 2

Prep Time: 8–10 minutes

Cook Time: 20 minutes

Nutritional Facts Per Serving (½ recipe):

Calories: 366

Fat: 17 g

Total Carbohydrate: 29 g

Protein: 24 g

Sodium: 340 mg

Ingredients:

- 2 salmon fillets (4 oz each)
- 1 tbsp green curry paste
- ½ cup low-sodium chicken broth
- 6 oz fresh green beans, trimmed
- ½ tsp toasted sesame seeds
- ½ cup light coconut milk
- ½ cup uncooked instant brown rice
- a pinch of pepper
- ½ tsp sesame oil
- lime wedges to serve

Directions:

1. Preheat the oven to 400 °F. Put the salmon into a baking dish. Add curry paste and coconut milk to a bowl and drizzle over the salmon.
2. Place the baking dish in the oven for 2 minutes or until the fish is cooked.
3. In the meantime, place rice, pepper, and broth in a saucepan. Stir well. Cover the saucepan and cook on medium heat for about 5 minutes.
4. Pour an inch of water into a saucepan and place it over medium heat. Place a steamer basket in the saucepan and the green beans in the steamer basket. Steam until the beans are crisp as well as tender

5. Transfer the beans to a bowl. Add sesame oil and sesame seeds and toss well.

6. To serve, divide the rice into two plates. Place a salmon fillet on each plate. Divide the beans among the plates. Drizzle coconut milk mixture on top and serve.

Shrimp and Grits

Time: 30 minutes

Serving Size: 2

Prep Time: 10 minutes

Cook Time: 20 minutes

Nutritional Facts Per Serving (¼ cup of grits with 1 cup of toppings):

Calories: 199

Fat: 7 g

Total Carbohydrate: 17 g

Protein: 17 g

Sodium: 637 mg

Ingredients:

For grits

¾ cup chicken broth, unsalted

¾ tsp butter

¼ cup grits (do not use degerminated grits)

For toppings

¾ tsp olive oil

1 small clove of garlic, minced

1 tbsp red or green bell pepper, diced

2 ½ tbsp whole pimento-stuffed green olives, sliced

½ tbsp capers

black pepper to taste

- lemon wedges to serve
- ½ bunch of green onions, chopped
- ½ tbsp sun-dried tomatoes in oil (but pat with paper towels to remove oil)
- ½ lb peeled, deveined shrimp
- 1 ¼ tbsp black olives, sliced
- ½ tbsp crumbled goat cheese
- ½ tbsp chopped parsley

Directions:

1. Pour broth into a saucepan and place it over medium-high heat. When the broth starts boiling, add grits and stir.

2. Bring the heat to medium-low and cook covered for about 10–12 minutes or until thick. Stir on and off. Turn off the heat.

3. Add butter and stir. Keep the bowl covered in a warm oven.

4. Pour oil into a skillet and let it heat over medium heat. When the oil is hot, add green onions, sun-dried tomatoes, and garlic and mix well. Cook until vegetables are slightly tender.

5. Add shrimp and green pepper and stir on and off until the shrimp are cooked. Stir in the olives and capers. Turn off the heat.

6. Divide the grits into two plates. Place a cup of the shrimp toppings over the grits. Garnish with goat cheese, cracked pepper, lemon wedges, and parsley and serve.

One-Pot Garlicky Shrimp and Spinach

Time: 25 minutes

Serving Size: 2

Prep Time: 10 minutes

Cook Time: 15 minutes

Nutritional Facts Per Serving (1 cup):

Calories: 226

Fat: 11.6 g

Total Carbohydrate: 6.1 g

Protein: 26.4 g

Sodium: 444 mg

Ingredients:

- 1 ½ tbsp extra-virgin olive oil, divided
- ½ lb spinach, chopped
- ¾ tsp grated lemon zest
- ½ lb shrimp, peeled, deveined
- ½ tbsp chopped parsley
- 3 medium garlic cloves, peeled, sliced, divided
- ⅛ tsp plus a tiny pinch of salt, divided
- ½ tbsp lemon juice
- ⅛ tsp crushed red pepper

Directions:

1. Pour ½ tbsp of oil into a pot and let it heat over medium heat. When the oil is hot, add half of the garlic slices and stir until light brown.

2. Stir in spinach and ⅛ tsp of salt and mix well. Cook until the spinach turns limp. Add lemon juice and stir. Remove the spinach mixture into a bowl.

3. Turn up the heat to medium-high heat.

Pour the remaining oil into the pot. When the oil is hot, add the rest of the garlic and stir. Cook until the garlic is light brown. Stir in the shrimp, the rest of the salt, and crushed red pepper.

4. Cook for a few minutes until the shrimp are pink. Stir on and off.

5. To assemble, divide the spinach into two plates.

6. Divide the shrimp and place it over the spinach.

7. Garnish with parsley and lemon zest and serve.

Chapter 11: Poultry

Turkey and Broccoli Crepe

me: 17 minutes

rving Size: 2

ep Time: 5 minutes

ok Time: 10–12 minutes

tritional Facts Per Serving (1 filled pe):

ories: 223

7 g

l Carbohydrate: 23 g

ein: 17 g

ium: 200 mg

redients:

1 cup broccoli, chopped

2 oz low-sodium turkey breast slices

2 prepackaged crepes (8 inches each)

4 cup shredded low-fat Colby Jack heese

ections:

Preheat the oven to 350 °F. Prepare a aking dish by greasing it with cooking pray.

Pour an inch of water into a saucepan nd place it over medium heat. Place a teamer basket in the saucepan and the roccoli in the steamer basket. Cover he saucepan. Steam until the broccoli is right green, crisp, as well as tender.

Warm the crepes following the

instructions on the package.

4. Divide the turkey slices, broccoli, and cheese equally and place them over the crepes.

5. Roll the crepes and place them in the prepared baking dish with the seam side facing down. Place the baking dish in the oven and set the timer for about 5–8 minutes or until heated through and the cheese melts.

Turkey or Chicken Casserole Over Toast

Time: 25 minutes

Serving Size: 2

Prep Time: 5 minutes

Cook Time: 15–20 minutes

Nutritional Facts Per Serving (1 slice of toast and ½ chicken casserole):

Calories: 236

Fat: 4 g

Total Carbohydrate: 23 g

Protein: 27 g

Sodium: 237 mg

Ingredients:

- ¾ cup low-sodium chicken broth
- 3 tbsp diced onions
- 1 cup cooked, cubed chicken or turkey
- 1 ½ tbsp white wine
- 1 tbsp chopped fresh rosemary

- 2 slices whole wheat bread, toasted
- ¼ cup diced celery
- ¼ green bell pepper, deseeded, chopped
- 1 ½ tbsp all-purpose flour
- ¼ cup chopped fresh parsley
- pepper to taste

Directions:

1. Pour 2 tbsp of broth into a nonstick pan and let it heat over medium-high heat. When the broth is hot and simmering, drop the vegetables into the pan and stir. Cook until they turn crisp as well as tender.
2. Turn down the heat to low. Place chicken in a bowl. Sprinkle flour over the chicken and toss lightly. Transfer the chicken to the pan with vegetables and stir. Let it cook for about 4–5 minutes.
3. Turn up the heat to medium-high. Add wine, herbs, pepper, and the rest of the broth. Mix well. Let it simmer until the sauce is a bit thick.
4. Spread half the chicken mixture over each toast and serve immediately.

Honey-Crusted Chicken

Time: 35 minutes

Serving Size: 4

Prep Time: 10 minutes

Cook Time: 25 minutes

Nutritional Facts Per Serving (1 chicken breast):

Calories: 224

Fat: 4 g

Total Carbohydrate: 20 g

Protein: 27 g

Sodium: 204 mg

Ingredients:

- 16 saltine crackers (2 square inches each) crushed
- 4 boneless, skinless chicken breasts (4 o each)
- 2 tsp paprika
- 8 tsp honey

Directions:

1. Preheat the oven to 375 °F. Spray some cooking spray into a baking dish.
2. Combine crackers and paprika in a bo Combine chicken and honey in anoth bowl. Dredge the chicken in crackers place it in the baking dish.
3. Place the baking dish in the oven and the timer for 20–25 minutes or until t chicken is well cooked inside and ligh brown or brown on the outside.
4. Serve hot.

Chicken Paella

Time: 48 minutes

Serving Size: 2

Prep Time: 5–8 minutes

Cook Time: 30–40 minutes

Nutritional Facts Per Serving (½ recipe):

Calories: 369

at: 6 g

otal Carbohydrate: 46 g

otein: 35 g

odium: 182 mg

ngredients:

- ½ tsp extra-virgin olive oil

- 1 leek (white part), thinly sliced

- ½ lb skinless, boneless chicken breast, cut into thin slices crosswise

- ½ red bell pepper, sliced & ½ tsp dried tarragon

- ½ cup frozen peas & 2 lemon wedges to serve

- ½ small onion, sliced

- 2 garlic cloves, minced

- 1 large tomato, chopped

- ⅓ cup brown rice

- 1 cup fat-free, unsalted chicken broth

- ⅛ cup chopped fresh parsley

rections:

Pour oil into a nonstick pan and let it heat over medium heat. When the oil is hot, add onion, garlic, chicken, and leeks and mix well. Cook for a few minutes until the chicken turns light brown.

Stir in bell pepper and tomatoes and cook for a few minutes. Stir in the rice, broth, and tarragon. When the mixture starts boiling, turn down the heat and cook covered for about 10 minutes. Add peas and mix well. Cook without the lid until the rice is soft. Stir on and off.

Distribute the paella onto two plates. Sprinkle parsley on top. Place a lemon wedge on each plate and serve.

Balsamic Roast Chicken

Time: 30 minutes

Serving Size: 4

Prep Time: 5 minutes

Cook Time: 20–25 minutes for every pound of chicken

Nutritional Facts Per Serving (¼ chicken):

Calories: 301

Fat: 13 g

Total Carbohydrate: 3 g

Protein: 43 g

Sodium: 131 mg

Ingredients:

- 1 small whole chicken (about 2 lb), skin loosened from the meat

- 2 small garlic cloves, finely minced

- freshly ground black pepper to taste

- ¼ cup balsamic vinegar

- 1 sprig rosemary

- ½ tbsp minced fresh rosemary or ½ tsp dried rosemary

- ½ tbsp olive oil

- 4 sprigs of fresh rosemary

- ½ tsp brown sugar

Directions:

1. Preheat the oven to 350 °F.

2. Rub oil on the meat beneath the skin. Combine garlic and rosemary in a bowl and rub it over the meat beneath the skin. Season with pepper. Place a rosemary sprig inside the cavity. Now tie the legs to the body with kitchen twine and place it in a roasting pan.

3. Place the pan in the oven and bake until the internal temperature of the meat in the thickest part shows 165 °F on the meat thermometer. Baste the chicken on and off with the juices that are in the pan.

4. Place chicken on a serving platter. Let it rest for a couple of minutes.

5. Meanwhile, add brown sugar and balsamic vinegar into a saucepan and place it over medium heat. Stir until the sugar melts and turn off the heat. It should not boil.

6. Slice the chicken and discard the skin. Drizzle the balsamic vinegar mixture over the chicken and serve garnished with rosemary.

BBQ Chicken Pizza

Time: 12 minutes

Serving Size: 2

Prep Time: 5 minutes

Cook Time: 5–7 minutes

Nutritional Facts Per Serving (2 wedges):

Calories: 261

Fat: 7 g

Total Carbohydrate: 28 g

Protein: 21 g

Sodium: 475 mg

Ingredients:

- ½ cup unsalted tomato sauce
- ½ green bell pepper, cut into thin rings
- ½ cup sliced mushrooms
- 2 tbsp BBQ sauce
- 1 thin whole-grain pizza crust (6 oz)
- ½ tomato, cut into thin round slices
- 2 oz cooked chicken breast, trimmed of fat, cut into 1-inch thick slices
- ½ cup shredded, low-fat mozzarella cheese

Directions:

1. Preheat the oven to 400 °F.

2. Spoon the tomato sauce over the pizza and spread it evenly. Place tomato, pepper, chicken, and mushroom slices all over the sauce. Trickle BBQ sauce over the toppings. Finely sprinkle cheese on top and place it in the oven.

3. Bake for a few minutes until the cheese melts.

4. Cut into four equal wedges and serve.

Chapter 12: Red Meat Recipes

Lasagna

Time: 1 hour 5 minutes

Serving Size: 4

Prep Time: 5 minutes

Cook Time: 60 minutes

Nutritional Facts Per Serving (¼ recipe):

Calories: 425

Fat: 13 g

Total Carbohydrate: 42 g

Protein: 33 g

Sodium: 500 mg

Ingredients:

1 medium onion, chopped

4 oz canned unsalted tomato sauce

3 oz unsalted tomato paste

1 ¾ cups water & ½ cup low-fat cottage cheese

5 oz dry lasagna noodles

1 ½ cups low-fat mozzarella cheese, shredded

½ lb extra-lean ground beef

¼ tsp dried basil

½ tsp garlic powder

½ tsp dried oregano

Directions:

Preheat the oven to 325 °F. Spray some cooking spray into a baking dish.

For preparing the sauce, cook beef and onion in a saucepan over medium heat until the beef is brown. Break the meat as you stir. Drain the excess fat from the pan.

3. Stir in the herbs, garlic powder, water, tomato paste, and sauce. When it starts boiling, turn down the heat and simmer for 5–7 minutes. Turn off the heat.

4. Spread a thin layer of sauce on the bottom of the prepared baking dish. Spread a layer of lasagna noodles. Spread some of the sauce over the noodles. Scatter cottage cheese and ½ cup mozzarella over the noodles.

5. Repeat the layers until all the ingredients are assembled in the baking dish. Cover the dish with aluminum foil.

6. Place the dish in the oven and set the timer for 50–60 minutes or until the noodles are cooked. Uncover and cook for about 5 minutes until the top is light brown.

7. Cut into four equal portions and serve.

Shepherd's Pie

Time: 1 hour 15 minutes

Serving Size: 3

Prep Time: 12–15 minutes

Cook Time: 50–60 minutes

Nutritional Facts Per Serving (1 ½ cups):

Calories: 258

Fat: 7 g

Total Carbohydrate: 19 g

Protein: 29 g

Sodium: 413 mg

Ingredients:

- ¼ lb ground turkey breast
- ½ lb lean ground beef
- ¼ cup chopped carrots
- ½ tsp olive oil
- ½ tbsp tomato paste
- ½ tsp finely chopped fresh thyme
- ½ tsp finely chopped fresh rosemary
- ⅛ tsp pepper
- ¼ tsp plus ⅛ tsp kosher salt
- 1 cup chicken stock
- ¼ cup frozen corn, thawed
- ¼ cup frozen peas, thawed
- ½ cup skim milk
- ½ tbsp butter
- 1 medium russet potato, cut into ¾-inch cubes
- ¼ cup chopped onions

Directions:

1. Cook potato cubes in a small pot of water, place them over high heat, and cook until they are soft.

2. Meanwhile, pour oil into a skillet and heat over medium heat. Once the oil is hot, add onions and carrots and cook until soft. Stir in the meat and cook until brown. As you stir, break the meat into smaller pieces. Stir in ¼ tsp salt, pepper, tomato paste, and herbs.

3. Pour stock and stir. When the mixture starts boiling, add peas and corn and cook

until dry.

4. Transfer the vegetable and meat mixtur into a casserole dish. Spread it evenly.

5. Preheat the oven to 400 °F.

6. Pour the potatoes into a colander. Plac the drained potatoes in the pot. Stir in milk, butter, and ⅛ tsp of salt. Mash the potatoes with an electric hand mixer o masher until smooth. Turn off the heat.

7. Spoon the mashed potatoes over the m and spread it evenly.

8. Place the casserole dish in the oven and set the timer for 20–25 minutes or unt slightly golden brown on top.

Beef Brisket

Time: 2 hours 35 minutes

Serving Size: 4

Prep Time: 5 minutes

Cook Time: 2–2 hours 30 minutes

Nutritional Facts Per Serving (3 oz meat with 3 oz of sauce):

Calories: 229

Fat: 9 g

Total Carbohydrate: 6 g

Protein: 31 g

Sodium: 184 mg

Ingredients:

- 1 medium onion, chopped
- ½ tbsp olive oil
- coarsely ground pepper to taste
- ½ can (from a 14.5 oz can) of choppe tomatoes with liquid, unsalted
- ½ cup low-sodium beef stock or red

- 1 ¼ lb beef brisket, trimmed of fat, cut into four equal pieces
- 2 garlic cloves, peeled, smashed
- ½ tsp dried thyme
- 2 tbsp red wine vinegar

Directions:

1. Pour oil into a Dutch oven and let it heat over medium-high heat.
2. Sprinkle salt and pepper over the brisket and place it in the Dutch oven. Cook until the meat is dark brown all over.
3. Remove the meat with a slotted spoon and place it on a plate lined with paper towels.
4. Add onions and sauté until brown. Stir in garlic and thyme and sauté until fragrant. Stir in the vinegar, tomatoes, and stock and boil. Turn off the heat.
5. Preheat the oven to 350 °F.
6. Place the beef back in the Dutch oven and place it in the oven. Set the timer for about 2 hours or roast until the meat is cooked.

Pork Tenderloin With Apples

Time: 28 minutes

Serving Size: 2

Prep Time: 5–8 minutes

Cook Time: 20 minutes

Nutritional Facts Per Serving (½ recipe):

Calories: 240

Fat: 6 g

Total Carbohydrate: 17 g

Protein: 26 g

Sodium: 83 mg

Ingredients:

- ½ tbsp olive oil
- freshly ground black pepper to taste
- 1 cup chopped apple
- ½ cup low-sodium chicken broth
- ½ lb pork tenderloin, fat trimmed
- 1 cup chopped onions
- 1 tbsp chopped fresh rosemary
- ¾ tbsp balsamic vinegar

Directions:

1. Preheat the oven to 450 °F. Spray some cooking spray into a baking pan.
2. Pour oil into a skillet and let it heat over high heat. Place the pork in the skillet. Sprinkle pepper over the pork. Turn the meat every minute or so and cook the pork until brown all over. Transfer the meat to the baking pan.
3. Shift the baking pan into the oven and set the timer for 15 minutes or until the internal temperature of the meat in the thickest part shows 165 °F on the meat thermometer.
4. Add apple and onion into the same skillet and cook for a couple of minutes. Stir in the rosemary. Cook until the apples are tender. Add broth and vinegar and mix well.
5. Turn the heat to high heat and cook until the sauce is thick. Turn off the heat.
6. Cut the meat into slices diagonally.

Distribute the pork onto two serving plates. Divide the apple sauce equally and spoon over the meat. Serve hot.

Beef Stroganoff

Time: 27 minutes

Serving Size: 2

Prep Time: 5 minutes

Cook Time: 20–22 minutes

Nutritional Facts Per Serving (2 ½ cups):

Calories: 273

Fat: 5 g

Total Carbohydrate: 37 g

Protein: 20 g

Sodium: 193 mg

Ingredients:

- ¼ cup chopped onions
- 2 cups uncooked, yolkless egg noodles
- ¼ cup water
- ¼ tsp paprika
- ¼ lb boneless beef round steak, cut into ¾-inch thick pieces, fat trimmed
- ¼ can fat-free cream of mushroom soup
- ½ tbsp all-purpose flour
- ¼ cup fat-free sour cream

Directions:

1. Cook onions in a pan over medium heat. When the onions are soft, stir in the beef and cook until brown and cooked inside.
2. Remove meat and onions with a slotted spoon and place in a bowl. Discard any cooked fat from the pan.
3. Cook the noodles following the directions given on the package.
4. Add cream of mushroom soup, flour, and water into a saucepan and whisk well. Place the saucepan over medium heat and keep stirring until the sauce is thick.
5. Add the meat into the saucepan along with paprika and mix well. Let it heat thoroughly.
6. Turn off the heat and stir in the sour cream.
7. Distribute the noodles into two bowls. Divide the meat mixture equally and spoon over the noodles. Serve.

Grilled Pork Fajitas

Time: 11 minutes

Serving Size: 4

Prep Time: 5 minutes

Cook Time: 5–6 minutes

Nutritional Facts Per Serving (1 fajita

Calories: 180

Fat: 3 g

Total Carbohydrate: 29 g

Protein: 17 g

Sodium: 382 mg

Ingredients:

- ½ tsp ground cumin
- ¼ tsp paprika & ⅛ tsp garlic powder
- ¼ tsp dried oregano
- ⅛ tsp ground coriander
- ½ lb pork tenderloin, cut into ½-inch

wide by 2 inches long strips

4 whole wheat tortillas (8 inches each)

1 ½ cups chopped tomatoes

½ cup salsa

¼ cup shredded sharp cheddar cheese

2 cups shredded lettuce

½ small onion, sliced

Directions:

You can use a grill or a broiler for cooking the pork, so choose the method that is suitable for you and preheat.

Add spices into a bowl and stir. Roll the pork strips in the spice mixture, so they are coated with it.

Lay the pork strips either in a cast-iron pan or grill basket. Place it in the grill or oven with broil mode at medium-high heat until brown. Flip the meat occasionally.

To assemble, divide the pork and onions equally and place them over the tortillas.

Divide the cheese, lettuce, tomatoes, and salsa among the tortillas.

Fold like a burrito and serve.

Chapter 13: Stew and Soup Recipes

Turkey Soup

Time: 1 hour 55 minutes (chilling time not included)

Serving Size: 5

Prep Time: 10 minutes

Cook Time: 1 hour 45 minutes plus chilling time

Nutritional Facts Per Serving (about 2 cups):

Calories: 178

Fat: 2 g

Total Carbohydrate: 25 g

Protein: 15 g

Sodium: 131 mg

Ingredients:

- Broth
- ½ turkey carcass
- 4 cups low-sodium chicken broth
- 2 cups water
- ½ onion, cut into 2 halves
- 1 ½ onion, chopped
- Soup
- ½ can (from a 14.1-oz can) of tomatoes, unsalted
- ¼ lb leftover light turkey meat, cut into bite-size pieces
- ½ cup rutabaga or turnip, peeled, diced
- 2 tbsp pearl barley, uncooked
- 2 carrots, peeled, cut into thin strips
- a pinch of dried thyme
- ½ onion, chopped
- ½ cup chopped celery
- ⅛ cup chopped fresh parsley
- 2 small bay leaves
- ½ can (from a 16 oz can) of white bean drained, rinsed
- black pepper to taste

Directions:

1. Firstly, make the stock: Place turkey carcass and quartered onion in a soup p Add water and broth and place the po over high heat. When it begins to boil turn down the heat and cook covered for about 30–45 minutes. Strain the st and discard the solids.

2. Place the strained stock in the refriger. for 6–8 hours. Discard any fat that is floating on top.

3. To make the soup, pour the chilled st into a soup pot. Add onion, celery, car thyme, pepper, tomatoes, turkey meat, rutabaga, parsley, bay leaves, pearl barle and white beans into the pot and brin the mixture to a boil over high heat.

4. Turn down the heat, let it boil gently, and cover it for 45–60 minutes. Stir occasionally.

5. Ladle the soup into soup bowls and se

Pumpkin Soup

Time: 17 minutes

Serving Size: 2

Prep Time: 5 minutes

Cook Time: 10–12 minutes

Nutritional Facts Per Serving:

Calories: 77

Fat: 1 g

Total Carbohydrate: 14 g

Protein: 3 g

Sodium: 57 mg

Ingredients:

6 tbsp water divided

½ can (from a 15-oz can) of pumpkin puree

¼ tsp ground cinnamon

pepper to taste & ⅛ tsp ground nutmeg

1 small green onion, green part only, chopped

½ small onion, chopped

1 cup vegetable broth, unsalted

½ cup fat-free milk

Directions:

Pour 2 tbsp of water into a saucepan and place it over medium heat. When the water is very hot, add onion and cook until the water has evaporated.

Stir in the pumpkin puree, broth, remaining water, cinnamon, and nutmeg. When it starts boiling, turn down the heat and let it boil gently for 4–5 minutes.

Add milk and heat for 2–3 minutes. Turn off the heat.

4. Ladle the soup into soup bowls. Top with green onions and pepper and serve.

Cream of Wild Rice Soup

Time: 55 minutes

Serving Size: 2

Prep Time: 10 minutes

Cook Time: 40–45 minutes

Nutritional Facts Per Serving (2 cups):

Calories: 236

Fat: 4 g

Total Carbohydrate: 38 g

Protein: 12 g

Sodium: 180 mg

Ingredients:

- ¾ tsp canola oil & ½ cup diced carrot
- 1 garlic clove, minced
- ½ tbsp minced parsley
- ½ tsp fennel seeds, crushed
- ½ cup unsalted canned or cooked white beans
- ¼ cup cooked wild rice
- 1 cup 1% milk & ¾ cup diced onion
- ½ cup diced celery
- ¾ cup chopped kale leaves
- 1 cup low-sodium vegetable stock
- ½ tsp ground black pepper

Directions:

1. Pour oil into a soup pot and let it heat over medium heat. When the oil is hot, add onion, celery, carrot, and garlic and

stir. Cook for a few minutes until the onion is light brown.

2. Add kale, stock, parsley, fennel, and pepper, and stir. Let it come to a boil.

3. Meanwhile, blend beans and milk in a blender until smooth. Pour the blended beans into the soup pot and stir. When it starts boiling, stir in the wild rice.

4. Turn down the heat and let it boil gently for about 20–25 minutes.

5. Ladle the soup into soup bowls and serve.

Tuscan White Bean Stew

Time: 1 hour 40 minutes

Serving Size: 3

Prep Time: 10 minutes plus soaking time

Cook Time: 90 minutes

Nutritional Facts Per Serving (1 ¼ cups stew with ⅓ croutons):

Calories: 307

Fat: 7 g

Total Carbohydrate: 45 g

Protein: 16 g

Sodium: 334 mg

Ingredients:

- Croutons
- ½ tbsp extra-virgin olive oil
- ½ slice whole-grain bread, cut into ½-inch cubes
- 1 garlic clove, quartered
- Soup
- 1 cup dried cannellini beans or any other white beans of your choice, rinsed, soaked

in water for 7–8 hours, drained

- ¼ tsp salt, divided
- 1 tbsp olive oil
- 2 medium carrots, peeled, cut into piece
- freshly ground pepper to taste
- ¾ cup vegetable broth or stock
- 3 cups water
- ½ bay leaf
- ½ cup chopped yellow onions
- 3 garlic cloves, chopped
- ½ tbsp chopped fresh rosemary plus 3 sprigs to garnish

Directions:

1. To make the soup, place white beans, b leaf, water, and ⅛ tsp salt in a soup pot and place the pot over high heat.

2. When it starts boiling, turn down the heat to low and cover the pot partially. Cook until the beans are soft. It can tak a long time.

3. Retain about 5–6 tbsp of the cooked water and drain off the rest. Transfer the beans to a bowl.

4. While the beans are cooking, pour oil into a pan and let it heat over medium heat. When the oil is hot, add garlic and cook for a few seconds until you get a pleasant aroma. Turn off the heat and le the garlic cool in the oil.

5. Discard the garlic and place the pan ov medium heat. Let the oil heat once aga stir in the bread cubes, and cook until light brown, stirring often. Turn off the heat.

6. Mash ¼ cup of the cooked beans and t

retained water until smooth.

Pour oil into the soup pot and let it heat over medium-high heat. When the oil is hot, add carrots and onions and cook until the carrots are crisp and tender.

Add garlic and stir-fry for a few seconds, and then add ⅛ tsp salt, chopped rosemary, and pepper and stir.

Add beans, mashed beans, and stock and stir. When it begins to boil, turn the heat low and let it come to a gentle boil. Turn off the heat.

Serve in bowls, topped with croutons and rig of rosemary.

White Chicken Chili

ne: 30 minutes

ving Size: 4

p Time: 10 minutes

k Time: 20 minutes

ritional Facts Per Serving (1 ½ s):

ories: 212

4 g

l Carbohydrate: 25 g

in: 19 g

um: 241 mg

redients:

can (from a 10-oz can) of white chunk hicken

can (from a 14.5-oz can) of low-odium diced tomatoes

medium onion, chopped

medium red bell pepper, chopped

- 1 small green bell pepper, chopped
- 3 garlic cloves, minced
- ½ tsp ground cumin
- 1 tsp chili powder
- ½ tsp dried oregano
- ¼ cup shredded low-fat Monterey Jack cheese
- 1 can (15 oz) low-sodium cannellini beans or any other white beans, rinsed, drained
- 2 cups low-sodium chicken broth or chicken stock
- cayenne pepper to taste
- 1 ½ tbsp chopped cilantro

Directions:

1. Pour oil into a soup pot and heat over medium-high heat. When the oil is hot, add garlic and onion and cook for a couple of minutes.

2. Stir in the bell peppers and cook for a couple of minutes.

3. Add spices and oregano and stir for a few seconds until you get a pleasant aroma.

4. Stir in beans, chicken, and broth. Lower the heat and cover the pot partially when it begins to boil. Cook until the vegetables are tender.

5. Ladle the chili into bowls. Serve garnished with cheese and cilantro.

Beef and Vegetable Stew

Time: 1 hour 25 minutes

Serving Size: 3

Prep Time: 10 minutes

Cook Time: 65–75 minutes

Nutritional Facts Per Serving (2 cups):

Calories: 216

Fat: 4 g

Total Carbohydrate: 24 g

Protein: 21 g

Sodium: 138 mg

Ingredients:

- ½ lb beef round steak, fat and gristle trimmed
- 1 cup diced onions
- ½ cup diced Roma tomatoes
- ¼ cup diced, unpeeled white potato
- ½ cup diced carrot
- ½ cup chopped kale
- 1 tsp canola oil
- ½ cup diced celery
- ¼ cup diced sweet potato
- ¼ cup diced mushrooms
- 2 garlic cloves, chopped
- ⅛ cup uncooked barley
- ½ tsp balsamic vinegar
- ½ tsp crushed dried sage
- ½ tbsp minced fresh parsley
- ½ tbsp dried oregano
- ½ tsp minced fresh thyme
- ½ tbsp dried oregano
- black pepper to taste
- 2 tbsp red wine vinegar
- 1 ½ cups low-sodium vegetable or beef broth

Directions:

1. Set the oven to broil mode and preheat the oven to medium heat. Place the me in a broiling pan and place it in the ove Cook for 12–14 minutes. Turn the mea over halfway through broiling. Make su not to overcook the meat.
2. Take the roasting pan out and let the meat rest until the vegetables are cook
3. Pour into a soup pot and let it heat ove medium-high heat. When the oil is hot, add vegetables and cook for a few minutes until the vegetables are slightl tender.
4. Stir in the barley. Let it cook for about minutes, stirring on and off.
5. Dry the meat with paper towels and c it into ½-inch cubes. Add meat, balsan vinegar, red wine vinegar, spices, stock and herbs, and mix well.
6. When the stew starts boiling, bring dc the heat. Let it cook for about 45–50 minutes or until the barley is soft and stew is thick.
7. Ladle into bowls and serve.

Salmon Chowder

Time: 26 minutes

Serving Size: 4

Prep Time: 5–6 minutes

Cook Time: 20 minutes

Nutritional Facts Per Serving (1 cup

alories: 166

at: 2.5 g

otal Carbohydrate: 26 g

otein: 11 g

dium: 207 mg

gredients:

¼ cup celery, chopped

1 cup low-sodium chicken broth

¼ cup frozen peas

1 small carrot, chopped

pepper to taste

½ tsp olive oil & 1 garlic clove, minced

1 ¼ cups frozen country-style hash browns with green pepper and onion

¼ tsp dill

3 oz pink salmon, boneless (from a pouch or can)

½ can (from a 15-oz can) cream-style corn, unsalted

6 oz of evaporated skim milk

rections:

Pour oil into a saucepan and heat over medium heat. Add celery and sauté for a few minutes when the oil is hot.

Add garlic and sauté until fragrant. Add hash browns, broth, peas, carrot, dill, and pepper and stir. When the mixture starts boiling, turn down the heat and simmer until the vegetables are tender.

Make pieces of salmon with a fork and add to the soup. Add evaporated milk and corn and stir. Heat thoroughly.

Ladle into soup bowls and serve.

Chapter 14: Snacks & Appetizer Recipes

Fresh Tomato Crostini

Time: 30 minutes

Size: 6 servings

Prep Time: 20 minutes

Cook Time: 10 minutes

Nutritional Facts Per Serving (1 crostini):

Calories: 150

Fat: 6 g

Total Carbohydrate: 19 g

Protein: 5 g

Sodium: 170 mg

Ingredients:

- 1 baguette, sliced into 1/2-inch-thick slices
- 2 cups cherry tomatoes, halved
- 1/4 cup fresh basil, chopped
- 1 garlic clove, minced
- 1 tbsp extra-virgin olive oil
- 1 tbsp balsamic vinegar
- 1/4 tsp salt
- 1/4 tsp black pepper
- 1/2 cup low-fat mozzarella, shredded

Directions:

1. Set your oven's temperature to 375 °F (190 °C).
2. Place the baguette slices in a single layer on a large baking sheet. Bake the bread for 8 to 10 minutes, or until just barely toasted. Remove from the oven and let the slices cool.
3. In a medium bowl, combine the cherry tomatoes, basil, garlic, olive oil, balsamic vinegar, salt, and pepper. Toss gently to combine.
4. Top each toasted baguette slice with a spoonful of the tomato mixture.
5. Sprinkle each crostini with a small amount of shredded low-fat mozzarella.
6. Bake the baking sheet once again in the oven for a further two to three minutes or until the cheese is melted.
7. Serve the fresh tomato crostini immediately, garnished with additional basil if desired.

Baked Brie Envelopes

Time: 45 minutes

Serving Size: 12 servings

Prep Time: 25 minutes

Cook Time: 20 minutes

Nutritional Facts Per Serving (1 envelope):

Calories: 150

Fat: 8g

Total Carbohydrate: 12g

Protein: 7g

Sodium: 220mg

Ingredients:

- 1 sheet whole-wheat phyllo dough, thawed

8 oz low-fat brie cheese, cut into 12 equal pieces

1/4 cup finely chopped walnuts

1/4 cup dried cranberries, chopped

1 tbsp honey

1/4 tsp ground cinnamon

2 tbsp melted unsalted butter

Cooking spray

Directions:

Turn on the oven to 375°F (190°C). Cooking spray should be used to coat a sizable baking sheet.

Lay out the thawed whole-wheat phyllo dough on a clean work surface. Cut the sheet into 12 equal squares.

In a small bowl, mix together the chopped walnuts, dried cranberries, honey, and ground cinnamon.

In the middle of each phyllo square, place a piece of brie cheese. Top the cheese with a spoonful of the walnut and cranberry mixture.

Gently fold the phyllo dough over the filling to create an envelope shape, making sure to enclose the cheese and filling completely. Use a bit of melted unsalted butter to seal the edges.

Transfer the brie envelopes to the prepared baking sheet. Lightly brush the top of each envelope with the remaining melted butter.

Bake the brie pouches in the oven for 18 to 20 minutes, or until the phyllo dough is crisp and golden brown.

Before serving, take the cooked brie envelopes out of the oven and allow them cool for a while.

Sweet and spicy snack mix

Time: 40 minutes

Serving Size: 16 servings

Prep Time: 10 minutes

Cook Time: 30 minutes

Nutritional Facts Per Serving (1/16 of the mix):

Calories: 130

Fat: 5g

Total Carbohydrate: 18g

Protein: 4g

Sodium: 110mg

Ingredients:

- 3 cups whole-grain cereal (such as Cheerios or Chex)
- 1 cup unsalted pretzel twists
- 1 cup unsalted dry-roasted peanuts
- 1 cup unsalted almonds
- 1/4 cup unsalted pumpkin seeds
- 2 tbsp unsalted butter, melted
- 2 tbsp honey
- 1 tbsp low-sodium soy sauce
- 1 tsp chili powder
- 1/2 tsp garlic powder
- 1/2 tsp onion powder
- 1/4 tsp cayenne pepper (optional)

Directions:

1. Preheat your oven to 300°F (150°C). Line a large baking sheet with parchment

paper or a silicone baking mat.

2. Combine whole-grain cereal, pretzel twists, dry-roasted peanuts, almonds, and pumpkin seeds in a large mixing bowl. Mix well.

3. In a separate small bowl, whisk together the melted unsalted butter, honey, low-sodium soy sauce, chili powder, garlic powder, onion powder, and cayenne pepper (if using).

4. Pour the butter and spice mixture over the cereal mixture. Stir gently until all the ingredients are evenly coated with the spice mixture.

5. Spread the snack mix onto the prepared baking sheet in an even layer.

6. Bake the snack mix for 30 minutes, stirring every 10 minutes to ensure even cooking.

7. Remove the snack mix from the oven and let it cool completely. Store the cooled snack mix in an airtight container for up to 1 week.

White bean dip

Time: 15 minutes

Serving Size: 8 servings

Prep Time: 15 minutes

Cook Time: 0 minutes

Nutritional Facts Per Serving (1/8 of the dip):

Calories: 100

Fat: 3g

Total Carbohydrate: 13g

Protein: 5g

Sodium: 120mg

Ingredients:

- 1 can (15 oz) cannellini beans, rinsed and drained
- 2 cloves garlic, minced
- 2 tbsp fresh lemon juice
- 2 tbsp extra-virgin olive oil
- 1/4 cup fresh parsley, chopped
- 1/2 tsp ground cumin
- 1/4 tsp paprika
- 1/4 tsp salt
- 1/4 tsp black pepper
- Whole-wheat pita chips, sliced vegetable or whole-grain crackers for serving

Directions:

1. In a food processor, mix the cannellini beans with the minced garlic, lemon ju extra virgin olive oil, chopped parsley, ground cumin, paprika, salt, and black pepper.

2. As necessary, scrape down the bowl's sides as you process the mixture until it becomes creamy and smooth. Add a tablespoon of water if the dip is too th until you get the appropriate consisten

3. Taste the dip and adjust the seasoning your preference.

4. Transfer the white bean dip to a servi bowl and garnish with additional pars or a sprinkle of paprika, if desired.

5. For a healthy and satisfying snack or appetizer, serve the white bean dip wi whole-wheat pita chips, sliced vegetal or whole-grain crackers.

Southwestern potato skins

Time: 60 minutes

Serving Size: 6 servings (2 potato skins per serving)

Prep Time: 15 minutes

Cook Time: 45 minutes

Nutritional Facts Per Serving (1 serving):

Calories: 180

Fat: 6g

Total Carbohydrate: 25g

Protein: 8g

Sodium: 220mg

Ingredients:

6 medium russet potatoes, scrubbed and dried

1 tbsp olive oil

1/2 tsp salt

1/4 tsp black pepper

1/2 cup cooked black beans, drained and rinsed

1/2 cup frozen corn, thawed

1/2 cup diced bell pepper (any color)

1/2 cup shredded low-fat cheddar cheese

1/4 cup chopped green onions

1/4 cup chopped fresh cilantro

1/2 cup plain low-fat Greek yogurt

1/2 cup salsa

Directions:

Turn on the oven to 400 °F (200 °C). A big baking sheet should be lined with aluminum foil.

Place the potatoes on the baking sheet after giving them many fork pricks. Bake for 45-50 minutes, or until the potatoes are tender when pierced with a fork. After taking them out of the oven, let them cool completely before handling.

3. Each potato should be split lengthwise. Scoop the meat from each potato half with a spoon, leaving a 1/4-inch-thick shell behind. Reserve the scooped-out potato flesh for another use, if desired.

4. Add salt and black pepper after brushing the potato skins with olive oil. When the edges are crispy, transfer the potato skins back to the baking sheet and bake for an additional 10 to 12 minutes.

5. Bell pepper, black beans, and corn should all be combined in a medium bowl. In each potato skin, spoon the bean mixture.

6. Sprinkle each potato skin with a small amount of shredded low-fat cheddar cheese. Bake the potato skins for an additional 3-5 minutes, or until the cheese is melted.

7. Remove the Southwestern potato skins from the oven and top with green onions and fresh cilantro.

8. Serve the potato skins with a dollop of low-fat Greek yogurt and a side of salsa for dipping.

Italian-style meatballs

Time: 55 minutes

Serving Size: 6 servings (4 meatballs per serving)

Prep Time: 20 minutes

Cook Time: 35 minutes

Nutritional Facts Per Serving (4 meatballs):

Calories: 230

Fat: 10g

Total Carbohydrate: 12g

Protein: 24g

Sodium: 320mg

Ingredients:

- 1 lb lean ground turkey
- 1/2 cup whole-wheat breadcrumbs
- 1/4 cup grated Parmesan cheese
- 1/4 cup fresh parsley, chopped
- 1/4 cup fresh basil, chopped
- 1 egg, beaten
- 2 garlic cloves, minced
- 1/2 tsp salt
- 1/4 tsp black pepper
- 1/4 tsp red pepper flakes (optional)
- 1 tbsp olive oil
- 2 cups low-sodium marinara sauce, warmed

Directions:

1. Preheat your oven to 375°F (190°C). Line a large baking sheet with parchment paper or a silicone baking mat.
2. In a large mixing bowl, combine the ground turkey, whole-wheat breadcrumbs, grated Parmesan cheese, chopped parsley, chopped basil, beaten egg, minced garlic, salt, black pepper, and red pepper flakes (if using). Mix the ingredients until well combined.
3. Using your hands, form the mixture into 24 meatballs, each about the size of a golf ball. Place the meatballs onto the prepared baking sheet, spacing them evenly apart.
4. In a large skillet, heat the olive oil over medium heat. Add the meatballs in batches, turning them frequently to brown all sides. Cook each batch for about 5-7 minutes, and then transfer the browned meatballs back to the baking sheet.
5. Place the baking sheet in the preheated oven and bake the meatballs for an additional 20-25 minutes, or until they are cooked through and no longer pink in the center.
6. Serve the Italian-style meatballs with warmed low-sodium marinara sauce on the side for dipping.

Black bean and corn quinoa

Time: 35 minutes

Serving Size: 6 servings

Prep Time: 15 minutes

Cook Time: 20 minutes

Nutritional Facts Per Serving (1 serving):

Calories: 220

Fat: 4g

Total Carbohydrate: 37g

Protein: 9g

Sodium: 180mg

Ingredients:

- 1 cup uncooked quinoa
- 2 cups low-sodium vegetable broth
- 1 cup of rinsed and drained canned bla

beans

1 cup thawed frozen corn kernels

1/2 cup diced red bell pepper

1/2 cup diced red onion

1/4 cup chopped fresh cilantro

1 lime, juiced

1 tbsp extra-virgin olive oil

1/2 tsp ground cumin

1/2 tsp chili powder

Salt and pepper to taste

...ections:

To get rid of any remaining bitterness, rinse the quinoa in a fine-mesh sieve with cold water.

Quinoa that has been rinsed and low-sodium vegetable broth go together in a medium saucepan. The mixture should be brought to a boil, then simmered for 15 to 20 minutes, covered, until the quinoa is cooked and has absorbed the stock.

After turning off the heat, leave the quinoa covered for five minutes. Using a fork, fluff the quinoa and set it aside to chill.

In a large mixing bowl, combine the cooled quinoa, black beans, corn, red bell pepper, red onion, and chopped cilantro. Mix well.

In a small bowl, combine the lime juice, extra virgin olive oil, cumin powder, chili powder, salt, and pepper. Pour the dressing over the quinoa mixture, then toss it.

To enable the flavors to merge, chill the black bean and corn quinoa for at least 30

minutes.

7. Serve the black bean and corn quinoa chilled or at room temperature.

Coconut shrimp

Time: 40 minutes

Serving Size: 4 servings

Prep Time: 20 minutes

Cook Time: 20 minutes

Nutritional Facts Per Serving (4 shrimp):

Calories: 230

Fat: 9g

Total Carbohydrate: 21g

Protein: 16g

Sodium: 300mg

Ingredients:

- 1 lb of peeled and deveined raw big shrimp
- 1/2 cup whole-wheat flour
- 1/2 tsp salt
- 1/4 tsp black pepper
- 2 large egg whites, beaten
- 1 cup unsweetened shredded coconut
- Cooking spray
- 1/2 cup low-sodium, low-sugar sweet chili sauce (for dipping, optional)

Directions:

1. Turn on the oven to 400 °F (200 °C). A sizable baking sheet should be lined with parchment paper and lightly sprayed with cooking spray.

2. In a shallow dish, mix together the whole-wheat flour, salt, and black pepper.

3. Place the beaten egg whites in another shallow dish.

4. Spread the unsweetened shredded coconut on a separate plate.

5. The shrimp should be dried with a paper towel. Each shrimp should be dredged in the flour mixture while being held by the tail and the excess should be shaken off. Then, dip the shrimp in the egg whites, allowing any excess to drip off. Finally, press the shrimp into the shredded coconut, making sure to coat both sides evenly.

6. Arrange the coated shrimp on the prepared baking sheet in a single layer. Lightly spray the shrimp with cooking spray.

7. Bake the coconut shrimp for 15-20 minutes, flipping them over halfway through cooking, or until the shrimp are cooked through and the coconut is golden brown.

8. The coconut shrimp should be removed from the oven and allowed to cool before serving. Provide low-sodium, low-sugar sweet chili sauce on the side for dipping the shrimp, if desired.

Orange juice smoothie

Time: 10 minutes

Serving Size: 2 servings

Prep Time: 10 minutes

Cook Time: 0 minutes

Nutritional Facts Per Serving (1

serving):

Calories: 175

Fat: 1g

Total Carbohydrate: 40g

Protein: 5g

Sodium: 30mg

Ingredients:

- 1 cup freshly squeezed orange juice
- 1/2 cup non-fat Greek yogurt
- 1 banana, sliced
- 1 cup frozen mango chunks
- 1/2 cup baby spinach leaves, washed and drained
- 1 tbsp chia seeds
- 1 tsp honey (optional)

Directions:

1. In a blender, combine the freshly squeezed orange juice, non-fat Greek yogurt, sliced banana, frozen mango chunks, baby spinach leaves, chia seeds and honey (if using).

2. Mix till smooth and creamy at high sp Add a little more orange juice or wate the smoothie is too thick to get the ri consistency.

3. Pour the smoothie into two glasses an serve immediately.

Berry and beet green smoothie

Time: 10 minutes

Serving Size: 2 servings

Prep Time: 10 minutes

Cook Time: 0 minutes

Nutritional Facts Per Serving (1 smoothie):

Calories: 190

Fat: 1g

Total Carbohydrate: 42g

Protein: 6g

Sodium: 100mg

Ingredients:

1 cup beet greens, washed and chopped

1 cup mixed berries (strawberries, blueberries, raspberries, and/or blackberries), fresh or frozen

1 medium banana, peeled and sliced

1 cup unsweetened almond milk

1/2 cup low-fat plain Greek yogurt

1 tbsp chia seeds

1 tbsp honey (optional)

Directions:

In a blender, combine the chopped beet greens, mixed berries, banana, unsweetened almond milk, low-fat plain Greek yogurt, and chia seeds.

When they are smooth and creamy, blend the ingredients at high speed. Add extra almond milk to the smoothie if it's too thick to get the right consistency.

Taste the smoothie and, if needed, add honey to sweeten it according to your preference.

Pour the smoothie into two glasses and serve immediately.

Mango and ginger smoothie

Time: 10 minutes

Serving Size: 2 servings

Prep Time: 10 minutes

Cook Time: 0 minutes

Nutritional Facts Per Serving (1 smoothie):

Calories: 190

Fat: 1g

Total Carbohydrate: 43g

Protein: 5g

Sodium: 50mg

Ingredients:

- 2 cups frozen mango chunks
- 1 cup low-fat plain yogurt
- 1/2 cup unsweetened almond milk
- 1 tbsp fresh ginger, peeled and grated
- 1 tbsp honey or agave syrup (optional)
- 1/4 tsp ground cinnamon
- A pinch of ground cardamom (optional)

Directions:

1. In a blender, combine the frozen mango chunks, low-fat plain yogurt, unsweetened almond milk, grated ginger, honey or agave syrup (if using), ground cinnamon, and ground cardamom (if using).

2. Until the smoothie is smooth and creamy, blend the ingredients at a high speed. To make sure all the ingredients are thoroughly incorporated, you might need to turn the blender off and scrape the sides with a spatula.

3. Taste the smoothie and adjust the sweetness by adding more honey or agave syrup if desired.

4. Pour the Mango and Ginger Smoothie into two glasses and serve immediately.

Pumpkin soup

Time: 50 minutes

Serving Size: 6 servings

Prep Time: 10 minutes

Cook Time: 40 minutes

Nutritional Facts Per Serving (1 serving):

Calories: 130

Fat: 3g

Total Carbohydrate: 23g

Protein: 4g

Sodium: 150mg

Ingredients:

- 2 tbsp olive oil
- 1 medium onion, chopped
- 2 garlic cloves, minced
- 4 cups pumpkin puree (fresh or canned)
- 4 cups low-sodium vegetable broth
- 1/2 cup low-fat milk or unsweetened almond milk
- 1/4 tsp ground nutmeg
- 1/4 tsp ground cinnamon
- 1/4 tsp ground ginger
- Salt and pepper, to taste
- Fresh parsley, chopped, for garnish

Directions:

1. In a big pot, warm the olive oil over medium heat. Add the chopped onion and cook for a further 3 to 4 minutes, o until it is soft and transparent.

2. For an additional minute, stir regularly t prevent burning after adding the mince garlic.

3. Add the low-sodium vegetable broth, nutmeg, cinnamon, and ginger after incorporating the pumpkin puree. The liquid should be brought to a boil, then simmer for 25 to 30 minutes with just occasional stirring.

4. Use an immersion blender or carefully transfer the soup to a blender to completely purée it. While blending soup, take cautious to let it cool slightly first and, if required, blend the soup in portions.

5. Stir the low-fat milk or unsweetened almond milk into the pureed soup befo adding it back to the saucepan. Add salt and pepper to taste when preparing the soup.

6. Warm the soup over low heat for anoth 5-10 minutes, stirring occasionally.

7. Serve the pumpkin soup hot, garnishe with fresh chopped parsley.

Fresh fruit smoothie

Time: 10 minutes

Serving Size: 2 servings

Prep Time: 10 minutes

Cook Time: 0 minutes

...tritional Facts Per Serving (1 ...ving):

...lories: 180

...: 1g

...al Carbohydrate: 43g

...tein: 3g

...ium: 40mg

...redients:

1 cup fresh strawberries, hulled

1 ripe banana, peeled and sliced

1/2 cup fresh blueberries

1/2 cup fresh pineapple chunks

1 cup baby spinach

1 cup low-fat Greek yogurt

1 cup ice cubes

1 tbsp honey (optional)

...ections:

...n a blender, combine the fresh ...trawberries, banana slices, blueberries, ...pineapple chunks, baby spinach, and low-...at Greek yogurt.

...Blend on high speed while adding the ...ce cubes until the mixture is smooth and ...reamy. You can add a small bit of water ...or milk to the smoothie to thin it down if ...t is too thick.

...Taste the smoothie and add honey if ...esired for added sweetness. Blend again ...or a few seconds to incorporate the ...oney.

...our the fresh fruit smoothie into two ...lasses and serve immediately.

Spicy Roasted Chickpeas

Time: 45 minutes

Serving Size: 6 servings

Prep Time: 5 minutes

Cook Time: 40 minutes

Nutritional Facts Per Serving (1/6 of the recipe):

Calories: 130

Fat: 4g

Total Carbohydrate: 18g

Protein: 6g

Sodium: 240mg

Ingredients:

- 2 cans (15 oz each) low-sodium chickpeas, drained and rinsed
- 1 tbsp olive oil
- 1/2 tsp smoked paprika
- 1/4 tsp cayenne pepper
- 1/4 tsp garlic powder
- 1/4 tsp onion powder
- 1/2 tsp salt

Directions:

1. Turn on the oven to 400 °F (205 °C). Using parchment paper, line a sizable baking sheet.

2. Dry the chickpeas thoroughly with a clean kitchen towel or paper towels.

3. Olive oil, smoked paprika, cayenne, garlic powder, onion powder, and salt should all be combined in a big bowl. Toss the chickpeas in the mixture to coat them evenly.

4. On the preheated baking sheet, distribute the chickpeas in a single layer.

5. Bake for 35-40 minutes, or until the chickpeas are golden brown and crispy, stirring every 10 minutes to ensure even roasting.

6. Remove from the oven and let the spicy roasted chickpeas cool slightly before serving.

Zucchini and Feta Stuffed Mushrooms

Time: 35 minutes

Serving Size: 4 servings (3 mushrooms per serving)

Prep Time: 15 minutes

Cook Time: 20 minutes

Nutritional Facts Per Serving (3 stuffed mushrooms):

Calories: 100

Fat: 6g

Total Carbohydrate: 7g

Protein: 5g

Sodium: 180mg

Ingredients:

- 12 large white button mushrooms, stems removed and finely chopped
- 1 small zucchini, grated and squeezed to remove excess moisture
- 1/4 cup crumbled feta cheese
- 1/4 cup whole-wheat breadcrumbs
- 2 tbsp fresh parsley, chopped
- 1 garlic clove, minced
- 1 tbsp olive oil
- Salt and black pepper, to taste

Directions:

1. Set the oven's temperature to 375°F (190°C). A baking sheet should be greased or lined with parchment paper.

2. Combine the grated zucchini, feta chee[se], parsley, garlic, and sliced mushroom ste[ms] in a medium bowl. To taste, add salt an[d] black pepper to the food.

3. Spoon a little amount of the feta and zucchini filling into each mushroom ca[p.] Lightly press the filling into place.

4. Place the stuffed mushrooms on the baking sheet that has been prepared.

5. Drizzle the stuffed mushrooms with ol[ive] oil.

6. Bake for 18 to 20 minutes, or until the filling is browned and the mushrooms [are] soft.

7. Remove from the oven and let the zucchini and feta stuffed mushrooms c[ool] slightly before serving.

Zesty Lemon Chickpea Salad

Time: 20 minutes

Serving Size: 6 servings

Prep Time: 15 minutes

Cook Time: 5 minutes

Nutritional Facts Per Serving (1 serving):

Calories: 170

Fat: 6g

Total Carbohydrate: 23g

Protein: 8g

dium: 150mg

gredients:

2 cups canned low-sodium chickpeas, drained and rinsed

1 cup cherry tomatoes, halved

1/2 cup diced cucumber

1/4 cup finely chopped red onion

1/4 cup chopped fresh parsley

2 tbsp extra-virgin olive oil

2 tbsp fresh lemon juice

1 garlic clove, minced

1/2 tsp ground cumin

Salt and black pepper, to taste

rections:

In a large bowl, combine the chickpeas, cherry tomatoes, cucumber, red onion, and parsley.

Mix the extra virgin olive oil, fresh lemon juice, minced garlic, ground cumin, salt, and black pepper in a separate small bowl.

Mix the chickpea salad thoroughly after adding the dressing.

Serve immediately or refrigerate for at least 30 minutes to allow the flavors to meld.

Roasted Red Pepper Hummus

ne: 15 minutes

ving Size: 8 servings

p Time: 15 minutes

ok Time: 0 minutes

Nutritional Facts Per Serving (1 serving):

Calories: 100

Fat: 5g

Total Carbohydrate: 12g

Protein: 4g

Sodium: 90mg

Ingredients:

- 1 (15 oz) can low-sodium chickpeas, drained and rinsed
- 1/2 cup jarred roasted red peppers, drained
- 3 tbsp tahini
- 2 tbsp extra-virgin olive oil
- 2 tbsp fresh lemon juice
- 1 garlic clove, minced
- 1/2 tsp ground cumin
- Salt and black pepper, to taste
- Fresh parsley and paprika, for garnish (optional)

Directions:

1. Combine the chickpeas, roasted red peppers, tahini, extra virgin olive oil, fresh lemon juice, minced garlic, ground cumin, salt, and black pepper in a food processor or blender.

2. Process the mixture until smooth and creamy, stopping to scrape down the sides as necessary.

3. Taste and adjust the seasoning as desired.

4. Place the hummus in a serving bowl and, if preferred, top with paprika and fresh parsley.

5. Serve with an assortment of fresh

vegetables, whole-grain crackers, or pita chips for dipping.

Spinach and Artichoke Stuffed Mushrooms

Time: 40 minutes

Serving Size: 6 servings

Prep Time: 20 minutes

Cook Time: 20 minutes

Nutritional Facts Per Serving (1 stuffed mushroom):

Calories: 80

Fat: 4g

Total Carbohydrate: 7g

Protein: 5g

Sodium: 150mg

Ingredients:

- 12 large white button mushrooms, stems removed and finely chopped
- 1 tbsp olive oil
- 1/4 cup onion, finely chopped
- 1 garlic clove, minced
- 1 cup fresh spinach, chopped
- 1/2 cup canned artichoke hearts, drained and chopped
- 1/4 cup low-fat cream cheese
- 1/4 cup grated Parmesan cheese
- 1/4 tsp salt
- 1/4 tsp black pepper

Directions:

1. Set the oven's temperature to 350°F (175°C). Use parchment paper to cover baking sheet.
2. Heat the olive oil in a medium skillet over medium heat. Add the onion and simmer for about 4 minutes, or until tender.
3. One minute later, add the garlic and continue cooking.
4. One minute later, add the garlic and continue cooking.
5. Add the spinach, artichoke hearts, and chopped mushroom stems after stirring. Simmer for about 5 minutes, or until the mushroom stems are soft and the spinach has wilted.
6. Stir in the low-fat cream cheese, freshly grated Parmesan cheese, salt, and pepper after turning off the heat in the skillet.
7. Spoon some of the spinach and artichoke mixture into each mushroom cap. Put the stuffed mushrooms on the baking sheet that has been prepared.
8. Bake the mushrooms for 20 minutes, or until they are cooked through and the filling is golden.
9. Remove from the oven and serve immediately.

Edamame and Avocado Dip

Time: 15 minutes

Serving Size: 8 servings

Prep Time: 15 minutes

Cook Time: 0 minutes

Nutritional Facts Per Serving (1/4 cu

ories: 100

: 6g

al Carbohydrate: 7g

tein: 5g

ium: 80mg

redients:

2 cups shelled edamame, cooked and cooled

1 medium ripe avocado, peeled and pitted

1/4 cup fresh cilantro, chopped

2 tbsp lime juice

1 garlic clove, minced

1/4 tsp ground cumin

1/4 tsp salt

2 tbsp water

2 tbsp extra-virgin olive oil

ections:

n a food processor, combine the cooked
edamame, avocado, cilantro, lime juice,
arlic, ground cumin, and salt. Blend until
mooth.

Once the dip has reached the appropriate
onsistency, add the water and olive oil
radually while the food processor is
unning.

Transfer the edamame and avocado
ip to a serving bowl and garnish with
dditional cilantro, if desired.

erve with your favorite whole-grain
rackers, pita chips, or raw vegetables for
healthy and delicious snack or appetizer.

Roasted Cauliflower and White Bean Dip

Time: 50 minutes

Serving Size: 8 servings

Prep Time: 10 minutes

Cook Time: 40 minutes

Nutritional Facts Per Serving (1/4 cup):

Calories: 110

Fat: 4g

Total Carbohydrate: 15g

Protein: 5g

Sodium: 160mg

Ingredients:

- 1 medium cauliflower head, divided into florets

- 2 tbsp extra-virgin olive oil, divided

- 1/2 tsp salt, divided

- 1/4 tsp black pepper, divided

- 1 can (15 oz) low-sodium cannellini beans, drained and rinsed

- 2 garlic cloves, minced

- 2 tbsp lemon juice

- 1/4 cup fresh parsley, chopped

- 1/4 cup grated Parmesan cheese

- Whole-grain crackers or raw vegetables, for serving

Directions:

1. Turn on the oven to 400 °F (200 °C). Use parchment paper to cover a baking sheet.

2. Cauliflower florets should be mixed with 1 tablespoon of olive oil, 1/4 teaspoon of salt, and 1/8 teaspoon of black pepper

in a sizable basin. On the baking sheet that has been prepared, distribute the cauliflower equally.

3. When roasting cauliflower, turn it occasionally to promote equal cooking and roast for 35 to 40 minutes, or until it is soft and golden brown.

4. In a food processor, combine the roasted cauliflower, cannellini beans, garlic, lemon juice, parsley, Parmesan cheese, remaining 1 tablespoon of olive oil, 1/4 teaspoon of salt, and 1/8 teaspoon of black pepper. Blend until smooth and creamy.

5. Place the dip in a serving bowl and, if wanted, top with more parsley and Parmesan cheese.

6. Serve the roasted cauliflower and white bean dip with whole-grain crackers or raw vegetables for a healthy and delicious appetizer.

Chapter 15: Bonus Chapter

Mediterranean Recipes
Mediterranean Grilled Salmon

Time: 14 minutes

Serving Size: 2

Prep Time: 5–6 minutes

Cook Time: 6–8 minutes

Nutritional Facts Per Serving (1 fillet):

Calories: 241

Fat: 10 g

Total Carbohydrate: 3 g

Protein: 28 g

Sodium: 143 mg

Ingredients:

⅛ cup chopped fresh basil

½ tbsp minced garlic & 2 salmon fillets (5 oz each)

2 green olives, chopped

½ tbsp chopped fresh parsley

1 tbsp lemon juice

cracked pepper to taste

2 thin lemon slices

Directions:

Preheat a grill or oven on broil mode to high heat. If you are using the grill, grease the grill rack with oil. If you are using the oven, grease the broiler pan with oil. Place the rack 4–6 inches below the heating element.

2. Add basil, parsley, garlic, and lemon juice to mix well. Place the fish fillets in the roasting pan and spray some cooking spray over the fish. Season the fish fillets with pepper.

3. Distribute equally the herb mixture and spread it over the fillets. If you are using the grill, place the herb side of the fish touching the grill grate.

4. Cook for 3–4 minutes. Flip sides and cook the other side for 3–4 minutes or until the fish flakes readily when pierced with a fork. The internal temperature of the fish in the thickest part should show 145 °F on the meat thermometer.

5. Top with olives and lemon slices and serve.

Mediterranean Chicken With Orzo Salad

Time: 40 minutes

Serving Size: 2

Prep Time: 10 minutes

Cook Time: 30 minutes

Nutritional Facts Per Serving (1 half of chicken breast with 1 cup salad):

Calories: 402

Fat: 7.5 g

Total Carbohydrate: 28.3 g

Protein: 32 g

Sodium: 512.7 mg

Ingredients:

- 1 skinless, boneless chicken breast (8 oz), halved
- ½ tsp grated lemon zest
- ¼ tsp pepper, divided
- 1 ½ tbsp extra-virgin olive oil
- ¼ tsp salt, divided
- 6 oz whole wheat orzo
- ½ cup chopped cucumber
- ⅛ cup chopped red onion
- 1 cup thinly sliced baby spinach
- ½ cup chopped tomatoes
- 1 tbsp chopped kalamata olives
- 2 small garlic cloves, peeled, grated
- ⅛ cup crumbled feta cheese
- 1 tbsp lemon juice
- 1 tsp chopped fresh oregano

Directions:

1. To make the chicken, preheat the oven to 425 °F.
2. Brush ½ tbsp of oil over the chicken. Season with half of each salt and pepper and put it into a baking dish.
3. Place the baking dish in an oven and bake until the chicken is cooked. It should take 20–25 minutes. To check if the chicken is cooked, insert a meat thermometer in the center of the thickest part of the meat. It should show 165 °F if the chicken is well cooked.
4. To make the salad, cook orzo following the directions on the package. Add spinach a minute before draining.
5. Combine orzo, cucumber, onion, tomato, olives, and feta cheese in a bowl.
6. To make the dressing, add olive oil, garli lemon juice, oregano, and the remaining salt and pepper in a bowl and whisk wel
7. Set aside about 2 tsp of the dressing and pour the rest into the salad bowl. Toss well.
8. Divide the salad among two plates. Plac half of the chicken breast on the salad o each plate.
9. Drizzle the remaining dressing over the chicken and serve.

Vegetable Hummus Bowl

Time: 35 minutes

Serving Size: 2

Prep Time: 10 minutes

Cook Time: 25 minutes

Nutritional Facts Per Serving (1 bowl

Calories: 360

Fat: 19 g

Total Carbohydrate: 39.5 g

Protein: 12.3 g

Sodium: 414.8 mg

Ingredients:

- ¾ cup cauliflower florets
- 1 garlic clove, peeled, thinly sliced
- ½ tsp dried oregano
- ½ medium red bell pepper, cut into 1-inch squares
- 1 tsp grated lemon zest & ½ cup humr
- ½ medium avocado, peeled, pitted, and chopped

1 cup cooked tricolored quinoa

lemon wedges to serve

¾ cup broccoli florets

½ tbsp extra-virgin olive oil

⅛ tsp salt

½ small zucchini, cut into 1-inch pieces

ections:

Preheat the oven to 425 °F.

Place cauliflower, garlic, and broccoli on a baking sheet. Pour oil over the vegetables. Add salt and oregano. Mix well and spread it evenly.

Place the baking sheet in the oven and set the timer for 10 minutes. Stir in the zucchini and bell pepper and spread it once again. Place the baking sheet in the oven and roast for 10–15 minutes or until the vegetables are crisp, tender, and light brown.

To assemble, distribute the vegetables into two bowls. Distribute equally the quinoa among the bowls. Top with ¼ cup of hummus in each bowl. Serve with lemon wedges and avocado.

arlic Roasted Salmon and Brussels Sprouts

e: 35 minutes

ving Size: 3

Time: 10 minutes

k Time: 25 minutes

ritional Facts Per Serving (⅓ pe):

Calories: 334

Fat: 15.4 g

Total Carbohydrate: 10.3 g

Protein: 33.1 g

Sodium: 485 mg

Ingredients:

- 6 large garlic cloves, halved
- 1 large garlic clove, minced
- 1 tbsp finely chopped fresh oregano, divided
- freshly ground pepper to taste
- 6 tbsp white wine
- lemon wedges to serve
- 2 tbsp extra-virgin olive oil
- ½ tsp salt, divided
- 3 cups brussels sprouts, trimmed, sliced
- 1 lb wild-caught salmon fillet, cut into three equal portions

Directions:

1. Preheat the oven to 450 °F.
2. Add minced garlic, oil, ¼ tsp salt, ½ tbsp oregano, and a little pepper into a bowl and stir.
3. Add halved garlic and brussels sprouts into a roasting pan and toss well. Add about 1 ½ tbsp of the garlic oil mixture and mix well. Spread it evenly in the pan and set the timer for 15 minutes. Stir the brussels sprouts halfway through roasting.
4. Add wine into the bowl with the remaining garlic oil mixture.
5. Take out the roasting pan and give the brussels sprouts a good stir. Lay the salmon over the brussels sprouts.

6. Pour the wine mixture all over the salmon and brussels sprouts. Scatter oregano on top. Sprinkle the remaining salt and some pepper and place them back in the oven.

7. Set the timer for about 10 minutes or until the salmon is cooked.

8. Serve salmon and brussels sprouts with lemon wedges.

Creamy Lemon Pasta With Shrimp

Time: 25 minutes

Serving Size: 2

Prep Time: 5 minutes

Cook Time: 20 minutes

Nutritional Facts Per Serving (1 ½ cups):

Calories: 403

Fat: 13.9 g

Total Carbohydrate: 45.5 g

Protein: 28.3 g

Sodium: 396.3 mg

Ingredients:

- 4 oz of whole wheat fettuccine pasta
- 6 oz peeled, deveined raw shrimp
- ½ tbsp finely chopped garlic & 2 cups loosely packed arugula
- ½ tsp grated lemon zest
- ⅛ tsp salt & ⅛ cup thinly sliced fresh basil
- ½ tbsp extra-virgin olive oil
- 1 tbsp unsalted butter
- ⅛ tsp crushed red pepper or to taste

- ⅛ cup plain yogurt
- 1 tbsp fresh lemon juice
- 3 tbsp grated Parmesan cheese plus ext to garnish

Directions:

1. Cook the fettuccine pasta following the directions given on the package. Retain about ¼ cup of the cooked pasta liquid and drain off the remaining.

2. In the meantime, place a nonstick skille over medium-high heat. Pour oil into the skillet. When the oil is hot, place th shrimp in the pan and cook until they turn pink. Stir on and off. The cooked shrimp will curl up and look pink in color. Remove the shrimp from the pa and place them in a bowl.

3. Turn the heat to medium heat and me butter in the same pan. When the butt melts, stir in the garlic and crushed rec pepper. Cook for a few seconds until aromatic. Make sure you do not burn red pepper.

4. Stir in the arugula and cook for about minute. Turn down the heat to low. St yogurt, pasta, retained cooked liquid, a lemon zest. Mix well.

5. Stir in the shrimp, salt, and lemon juic Turn off the heat. Add Parmesan chee and toss well.

6. Divide the pasta and shrimp into two plates. Garnish with basil and some Parmesan if using and serve.

Slow Cooker Recipes

Vegetarian Bolognese

Time: 2 hours 45 minutes

Serving Size: 4

Prep Time: 15 minutes

Cook Time: 2 hours 30 minutes

Nutritional Facts Per Serving (1 cup spaghetti with ¾ cup sauce):

Calories: 434

Fat: 12.6 g

Total Carbohydrate: 64.3 g

Protein: 15.9 g

Sodium: 411 mg

Ingredients:

½ can (from a 28-oz can) of diced tomatoes

¼ cup low-sodium vegetable broth or water

¼ cup chopped celery

1 ½ tbsp extra-virgin olive oil

½ tsp Italian seasoning

⅛ tsp ground pepper

¼ cup heavy cream

¼ cup grated Parmesan cheese

¼ cup dry white wine

½ cup chopped onion

¼ cup chopped carrot

1 tbsp minced garlic

¼ tsp salt

1 can (15 oz) unsalted cannellini beans or any other small white beans of your choice, drained, rinsed

½ lb whole wheat spaghetti

• ⅛ cup chopped fresh basil

Directions:

1. Place tomatoes, broth, celery, oil, Italian seasoning, pepper, wine, onion, carrot, garlic, and pepper in a slow cooker. Give it a good stir.

2. Close the lid and set it on high with a timer for 2 hours or on low with a timer for 4 hours.

3. Add beans and cream during the last 30 minutes of cooking.

4. Cook the spaghetti following the directions given on the package. Distribute the spaghetti into four serving bowls. Distribute the sauce equally and spoon over the spaghetti.

5. Sprinkle Parmesan and basil on top and serve.

Chicken Stew

Time: 2 hours 40 minutes

Serving Size: 5

Prep Time: 10 minutes

Cook Time: 2 hours 30 minutes

Nutritional Facts Per Serving (1 cup):

Calories: 180

Fat: 2 g

Total Carbohydrate: 18 g

Protein: 21 g

Sodium: 433.8 mg

Ingredients:

• 1 lb boneless, skinless chicken breasts cut into 1-inch cubes

- 1 ½ cups peeled, cubed potatoes
- ½ cup sliced celery
- ½ tsp paprika
- ¼ tsp rubbed sage
- ½ can (from a 6-oz can) of unsalted tomato paste
- 1 ½ tbsp cornstarch
- 1 can (from a 14.5-oz can) of reduced-sodium chicken broth
- ½ cup chopped onion
- ½ cup thinly sliced carrots
- ¼ tsp pepper
- ¼ tsp dried thyme
- ⅛ cup cold water
- shredded Parmesan cheese to garnish (optional)

Directions:

1. Add chicken, vegetables, herbs, broth, and spices into a slow cooker and stir.
2. Close the lid and set the cooker on high with a timer for 2 hours or until the chicken is cooked. Combine cornstarch with water and pour into the pot. Mix well and cook for another 30 minutes or until the stew is thick.
3. Serve garnished with Parmesan cheese if desired.

Chicken and Orzo With Tomatoes and Olives

Time: 3 hours 15 minutes

Serving Size: 8

Prep Time: 15 minutes

Cook Time: 2 ½–3 hours

Nutritional Facts Per Serving (1 ½ cups):

Calories: 278

Fat: 4.7 g

Total Carbohydrate: 29.5 g

Protein: 29.1 g

Sodium: 433.8 mg

Ingredients:

- 2 lb boneless, skinless chicken breasts, trimmed, cut into four equal portions
- 4 medium tomatoes, chopped
- zest of 2 lemons, grated
- juice of 2 lemons & 1 tsp salt
- 1 ½ cups whole wheat orzo
- 4 tbsp chopped fresh parsley
- 2 cups low-sodium chicken broth
- 2 medium onions, sliced
- 2 tsp herbes de Provence
- 1 tsp ground pepper
- ⅔ cup quartered black or green olives

Directions:

1. Place chicken, onions, herbes de Provence, lemon juice, lemon zest, pep and salt in a slow cooker and stir.
2. Pour broth all over the ingredients. Clo the lid and set the cooker on high with a timer for 1 ½ hours or on low for 3

hours.

Add orzo and olives and stir. Close the lid and cook for another 30 minutes until the orzo is al dente.

Give it a good stir. Garnish with parsley and serve.

Coconut–Red Curry Squash Soup

Time: 3 hours 10 minutes

Serving Size: 4

Prep Time: 10 minutes

Cook Time: 3 hours

Nutritional Facts Per Serving (1 ¼ cups):

Calories: 182

4 g

Total Carbohydrate: 35 g

Protein: 5 g

Sodium: 341 mg

Ingredients:

½ tbsp unsalted butter

½ tbsp olive oil

large onion, chopped

tsp minced garlic

tbsp minced fresh ginger

cups peeled, chopped butternut squash

medium potato, peeled and chopped

cups vegetable stock

½ tbsp red curry paste

tsp brown sugar

½ tsp salt

- ¼ tsp freshly ground black pepper
- 1 tbsp fresh lemon juice
- ½ can (from a 13.5-oz can) of light coconut milk
- 1 tbsp chopped fresh cilantro

Directions:

1. Add oil and butter into a skillet and place it over medium heat. Add onion, ginger, curry paste, and garlic and sauté for 2–3 minutes when the butter melts. Stir often until the onions are translucent. Transfer the onion mixture to the slow cooker.

2. Add butternut squash, potato, vegetable stock, brown sugar, salt, and pepper and give it a good stir.

3. Close the lid. Set the cooker on high with a timer for 3 hours or until the vegetables are soft. You can also cook on low for 6–7 hours.

4. Blend the soup in a blender or with an immersion blender until smooth. Add coconut milk and lemon juice and stir.

5. Ladle into soup bowls. Garnish with cilantro and serve.

Caribbean Pot Roast

Time: 4 hours 10 minutes

Serving Size: 3

Prep Time: 10 minutes

Cook Time: 4 hours

Nutritional Facts Per Serving (⅓ recipe):

Calories: 469

Fat: 30 g

Total Carbohydrate: 4 g

Protein: 43 g

Sodium: 582 mg

Ingredients:

- 1 tbsp vegetable oil or canola oil
- ½ jalapeño pepper, diced
- ¾ cup chopped red onion
- ½ tbsp brown sugar
- ¾ tsp dried oregano
- ½ tsp ground coriander
- ½ tbsp all-purpose flour
- ½ can (from a 15-oz can) of low-sodium tomato sauce
- 1 ½ lb boneless beef chuck roast
- 2 garlic cloves, chopped
- ½ tsp kosher salt
- ¾ tsp chili powder or to taste
- ¾ tsp ground cumin
- ⅛ tsp ground cinnamon
- zest of ½ orange, grated

Directions:

1. Pour oil into a skillet and place the skillet over medium-high heat. When the oil is hot, add beef roast and cook until brown. Transfer the meat to the slow cooker.

2. Add onion into the same skillet and cook for a couple of minutes. Stir in garlic and jalapeño. Cook until the onion turns pink. Add brown sugar, oregano, coriander, flour, salt, chili powder, cumin, and orange zest and mix well. When the sugar dissolves, add the tomato sauce and mix well.

3. Turn off the heat and spoon the sauce over and around the roast.

4. Close the lid and set it on low with a timer for 4 hours. Once cooked, take out the roast and place it on your cutti board. Let it cool for about 8–10 minu

5. Discard any fat that may be floating on top of the sauce.

6. Slice the roast and serve with sauce.

Air Fryer Recipes

Sweet Potato Tots

Time: 1 hour 20 minutes

Serving Size: 2

Prep Time: 20 minutes

Cook Time: 60 minutes

Nutritional Facts Per Serving (6 tots

Calories: 78

Fat: none

Total Carbohydrate: 19 g

Protein: 1 g

Sodium: 335 mg

Ingredients:

- 1 sweet potato (about 7 oz)
- a pinch of garlic powder
- 6 tbsp unsalted ketchup
- ½ tbsp potato starch
- ½ tsp plus ⅛ tsp kosher salt

Directions:

1. Boil some water in a small pot over h heat. Drop the sweet potato in the po

and boil until the sweet potato is tender and can be pierced easily with a fork.

2. Drain the water and place it aside to cool. Using the large holes of a box grater, grate the sweet potatoes.

3. Place sweet potato in a bowl. Sprinkle potato starch, ½ tsp salt, and garlic powder and mix well. Make 12 equal portions of the mixture and shape them into tots (sort of small cylindrical shape).

4. Preheat the air fryer to 400 °F. Grease the air fryer basket by spraying some cooking spray. Place the tots in the air fryer basket. Set the timer for 12–14 minutes or until light brown. Turn the tots over after about 6–7 minutes of cooking.

5. Place the sweet potato tots on a serving platter. Add the remaining salt to the ketchup. Serve tots with ketchup.

- ¼ tsp ground paprika
- ¼ tsp chili powder
- pepper to taste
- ¾ tbsp olive oil
- ¼ tsp parsley flakes
- ¼ tsp sea salt

Directions:

1. To cut the potato into ⅛, quarter the potato lengthwise. Cut each quarter into two lengthwise, so you will get eight wedges in all.

2. Preheat the air fryer to 400 °F.

3. Toss the potatoes with oil, parsley, and seasonings. Spread the potato wedges in the air fryer basket and set the timer for 15 minutes. Turn the wedges over every 5 minutes until it is cooked through inside and light brown outside.

Potato Wedges

Time: 20 minutes

Serving Size: 2

Prep Time: 5 minutes

Cook Time: 15 minutes

Nutritional Facts Per Serving (4 wedges):

Calories: 129

Fat: 5 g

Total Carbohydrate: 19 g

Protein: 2 g

Sodium: 230 mg

Ingredients:

1 medium russet potato, cut into 8 equal wedges

Italian–Style Meatballs

Time: 25 minutes

Serving Size: 6

Prep Time: 10 minutes

Cook Time: 10–15 minutes

Nutritional Facts Per Serving (2 meatballs):

Calories: 122

Fat: 8 g

Total Carbohydrate: 0 g

Protein: 10 g

Sodium: 254 mg

Ingredients:

- 1 tbsp olive oil
- ½ tbsp minced garlic
- 1 tbsp milk & 2.6 oz bulk turkey sausage
- ⅓ lb lean ground beef
- 1 small egg, lightly beaten
- ½ tbsp finely chopped fresh rosemary
- ½ tbsp Dijon mustard
- ½ medium shallot, minced
- ⅛ cup whole wheat panko breadcrumbs
- ⅛ cup finely chopped fresh flat-leaf parsley
- ½ tbsp finely chopped fresh thyme
- ¼ tsp kosher salt

Directions:

1. Preheat the air fryer to 400 °F.
2. Pour oil into a nonstick pan and let it heat over medium-high heat. When the oil is hot, stir the shallot into the oil. Cook for a couple of minutes.
3. Stir in garlic and cook for a few seconds until you get a nice aroma. Turn off the heat.
4. Place panko breadcrumbs in a bowl. Drizzle milk over it and stir. Let it soak for 5 minutes.
5. Stir in shallot, beef, sausage, garlic, egg, salt, mustard, and herbs.
6. Make 12 equal portions of the mixture and shape each portion into a ball. Lay the meatballs in the air fryer basket. Set the timer for about 10–12 minutes or until they are light brown. Turn the meatballs over after about 7–8 minutes of cooking.
7. You can serve it as an appetizer or simmer it in marinara sauce and serve it over whole wheat pasta, zucchini noodle or brown rice.

Fried Zucchini

Time: 30 minutes

Serving Size: 2

Prep Time: 10 minutes

Cook Time: 20 minutes

Nutritional Facts Per Serving (⅓ cup)

Calories: 64

Fat: 5 g

Total Carbohydrate: 5 g

Protein: 2 g

Sodium: 345 mg

Ingredients:

- 1 tbsp grated Parmesan cheese
- ¼ tsp dried oregano
- ⅛ tsp garlic powder
- ⅛ tsp pepper
- 1 large zucchini (around 8 inches), trimmed, cut into ¼-inch thick round slices
- ½ tbsp extra-virgin olive oil
- ¼ tsp salt
- ⅛ tsp onion powder
- a pinch of crushed red pepper or to tas
- 1 tsp lemon juice

Directions:

1. Preheat the air fryer to 400 °F.
2. Add oil, Parmesan, and spices into a bo

and stir. Sprinkle the Parmesan mixture over the zucchini slices.

Place the zucchini in the air fryer basket in a single layer. Set the timer for 10–12 minutes or until golden brown. Make sure to turn the zucchini slices over halfway through frying.

Place the fried zucchini on a serving platter. Drizzle lemon juice on top and serve.

Loaded Potatoes

me: 25 minutes

ving Size: 1

p Time: 10 minutes

ok Time: 15 minutes

tritional Facts Per Serving (4 atoes):

ories: 199

7 g

l Carbohydrate: 26 g

ein: 7 g

um: 287 mg

redients:

baby Yukon Gold potatoes (about 5.5 z in all)

center-cut bacon slice

tbsp finely shredded reduced-fat heddar cheese

tiny pinch of kosher salt

tsp olive oil

tbsp chopped fresh chives

tbsp reduced-fat sour cream

Directions:

1. Preheat the air fryer to 350 °F.

2. Drizzle oil over the potatoes and spread them in the air fryer basket. Set the timer for 25 minutes or cook until you can pierce the potato easily with a fork. Stir every 10 minutes.

3. Place bacon in a pan and place the pan over medium heat. Cook until crisp. Remove bacon with a slotted spoon and place it on a plate lined with paper towels. When it cools, crumble the bacon.

4. When the potatoes cool slightly, take one potato at a time and squeeze lightly, so it splits open. Place on a serving platter.

5. Trickle the cooked bacon fat over the potatoes. Garnish with chives, sour cream, cheese, and bacon. Serve right away.

Chapter 16: Meal Plan

Day 1

- *Breakfast:* Cinnamon rolls
- *Lunch:* Beet and orange salad
- *Snack or appetizer:* Baked brie envelopes
- *Dinner:* Yellow lentils with spinach and ginger

Day 2

- *Breakfast:* Vegan sweet potato waffles
- *Lunch:* Quinoa egg salad wrap
- *Snack or appetizer:* Fresh tomato crostini
- *Dinner:* BBQ chicken pizza

Day 3

- *Breakfast:* Nut and berry parfait
- *Lunch:* Buffalo chicken salad
- *Snack or appetizer:* Sweet and spicy snack mix
- *Dinner:* One-pot garlicky shrimp

Day 4

- *Breakfast:* Summer skillet vegetable and egg scramble
- *Lunch:* Rice Noodles with spring vegetables
- *Snack or appetizer:* White bean dip
- *Dinner:* Pork tenderloin with apples

Day 5

- *Breakfast:* Oat and nut breakfast bars
- *Lunch:* Turkey and broccoli crepe
- *Snack or appetizer:* Southwestern potato skins
- *Dinner:* Beef and vegetable stew

Day 6

- *Breakfast:* Chocolate chip bread
- *Lunch:* Chicken burritos
- *Snack or appetizer:* Italian-style meatball
- *Dinner:* Salmon and asparagus farro bo

Day 7

- *Breakfast:* Orange juice smoothie
- *Lunch:* Chicken salad
- *Snack or appetizer:* Black bean and corr quinoa
- *Dinner:* Creamed Swiss chard with hal and tomato salsa

Day 8

- *Breakfast:* Nut and berry parfait
- *Lunch:* Sloppy Joes
- *Snack or appetizer:* Coconut shrimp
- *Dinner:* Grilled pork fajitas

Day 9

Breakfast: Raspberry chocolate scones

Lunch: Turkey and broccoli crepe

Snack or appetizer: Orange juice smoothie

Dinner: Southwestern bowl

Day 10

Breakfast: Summer vegetable and egg scramble

Lunch: Pasta salad with dill

Snack or appetizer: White bean dip

Dinner: Creamy lemon pasta

Day 11

Breakfast: Cranberry orange muffins

Lunch: Quinoa egg salad wrap

Snack or appetizer: Baked brie envelopes

Dinner: Black bean and sweet potato rice bowls

Day 12

Breakfast: Raspberry chocolate scones

Lunch: Black bean and sweet potato rice bowls

Snack or appetizer: Berry and beet green smoothie

Dinner: Shepherd's pie

Day 13

Breakfast: Chocolate smoothie

Lunch: Mixed bean salad

Snack or appetizer: Fresh tomato crostini

- *Dinner:* Pasta primavera

Day 14

- *Breakfast:* Cranberry orange muffins
- *Lunch:* Chimichurri noodle bowls
- *Snack or appetizer:* Sweet and spicy snack mix
- *Dinner:* Beef brisket with cheesy baked zucchini

Day 15

- *Breakfast:* Oat and nut breakfast bar
- *Lunch:* White bean and veggie salad
- *Snack or appetizer:* Southwestern potato skins
- *Dinner:* Vegetable calzone with vegetable dip and potato wedges

Day 16

- *Breakfast:* Cinnamon rolls
- *Lunch:* Green curry salmon with green beans and brown rice pilaf
- *Snack or appetizer:* Coconut shrimp
- *Dinner:* Chicken and orzo with tomatoes and olives

Day 17

- *Breakfast:* Fresh fruit smoothie
- *Lunch:* Turkey soup
- *Snack or appetizer:* Sesame-crusted tofu
- *Dinner:* Turkey or chicken casserole over toast

Day 18

- Breakfast: Cinnamon rolls
- Lunch: Tuscan white bean stew
- Snack or appetizer: Mango and ginger smoothie
- Dinner: Lasagna with toasted whole wheat bread

Day 19

- *Breakfast:* Vegan sweet potato waffles
- *Lunch:* Quinoa egg salad wrap
- *Snack or appetizer:* Baked brie envelopes
- *Dinner:* Quinoa risotto with arugula and Parmesan with glazed radish

Day 20

- *Breakfast:* Whole-grain banana bread
- *Lunch:* Tuna pita pockets
- *Snack or appetizer:* Pumpkin soup
- *Dinner:* Beef stroganoff

Day 21

- *Breakfast:* Pumpkin pie smoothie
- *Lunch:* Chimichurri noodle bowls
- *Snack or appetizer:* Fresh tomato crostini
- *Dinner:* Black bean wrap

Day 22

- *Breakfast:* Southwestern cornmeal muffins
- *Lunch:* Cucumber and pineapple salad
- *Snack or appetizer:* Fresh fruit smoothie

- *Dinner:* Salmon chowder

Day 23

- *Breakfast:* Whole-grain banana bread
- *Lunch:* Creamy lemon pasta with shrimp
- *Snack or appetizer:* White bean dip
- *Dinner:* Chicken paella

Day 24

- *Breakfast:* Nut and berry parfait
- *Lunch:* White bean and veggie salad
- *Snack or appetizer:* Sweet and spicy snack mix
- *Dinner:* Balsamic roast chicken with braised kale and cherry tomatoes

Day 25

- *Breakfast:* Mango and ginger smoothie
- *Lunch:* White chicken chili
- *Snack or appetizer:* Pumpkin soup
- *Dinner:* Black bean and corn quinoa

Day 26

- *Breakfast:* Vegan sweet potato waffles
- *Lunch:* Cream of wild rice soup
- *Snack or appetizer:* Coconut shrimp
- *Dinner:* Caribbean pot roast

Day 27

- *Breakfast:* Oat and nut breakfast bars
- *Lunch:* Mediterranean chicken salad

Snack or appetizer: Orange juice smoothie

Dinner: Garlic roasted salmon and brussels sprouts

Day 28

Breakfast: Berry and beet green smoothie

Lunch: Vegetable hummus bowls

Snack or appetizer: Italian-style meatballs

Dinner: Beef and vegetable stew

Free Gift

Thank you! Discover your gift inside! Dive into a rich assortment of Mediterranean Diet Cookbook for Beginners recipes for added inspiration. Gift it or share the PDF effortlessly with friends and family via a single click on WhatsApp or other social platforms.
Bon appétit!

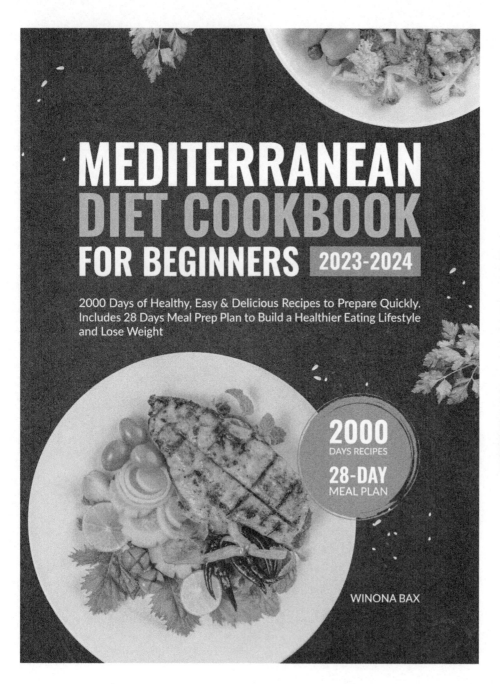

Chapter 17: Measurement Conversion Chart

.S. System	Metric
inch	2.54 centimeters
fluid ounce	29.57 milliliters
pint (16 ounces)	473.18 milliliters, 2 cups
quart (32 ounces)	1 liter, 4 cups
gallon (128 ounces)	4 liters, 16 cups
pound (16 ounces)	437.5 grams (0.4536 kilogram), 473.18 milliliters
ounces	2 tablespoons, 28 grams
cup (8 ounces)	237 milliliters
teaspoon	5 milliliters
tablespoon	15 milliliters (3 teaspoons)
Fahrenheit (subtract 32 and divide by 1.8 to get Celsius)	Centigrade (multiply by 1.8 and add 32 to get Fahrenheit)

Conclusion

Dietary Approaches to Stop Hypertension, also known as the DASH diet, is a unique dietary protocol designed to prevent or reduce hypertension. In recent decades, hypertension or high blood pressure has become a massive global concern. The usual course of action is to depend on pharmaceuticals. Alas, these pharmaceuticals also come with their own set of side effects and reactions. Therefore, focusing on a natural remedy or a holistic approach to improving your health is better. This is where your diet steps into the picture. The first step to tackling hypertension is to pay attention to your food choices. The diet you follow is one of the essential pillars of your overall health and well-being.

A typical Western diet is rich in sodium, processed foods, sugars, carbohydrates, unhealthy fats, and all things undesirable. It also lacks the essential nutrition your body requires to function effectively. If you cannot cater to your body's nutritional requirements, you cannot expect it to function as intended. The good news is that your diet is well within your control regardless of all that happens in your life. The DASH diet is the first step toward improving your health. It is a predominantly plant-based diet that increases the consumption of nutritious and wholesome fruits, whole grains, vegetables, and lean meats while reducing sodium consumption. Since high sodium intake is associated with an increased risk of blood pressure, reducing it is needed.

Following this diet can tackle high blood pressure levels and improve your overall health. From attaining your weight loss and fitness goals to reducing the risk of cardiovascular disorders and metabolic disorders, this is a wonderful diet. Your consumption of sugars, unhealthy fats, and processed foods will automatically reduce when you shift to the DASH diet. Once you become conscious of the foods you consume, you will notice an overall change in your well-being. However, you will need to be patient while making any dietary change. Even though it doesn't sound like much, it's a significant change for your body and mind. So you will need sufficient time to get accustomed to your new diet.

If you are eager to shift to this diet and reclaim control of your health, this book will act as your guide. This book has everything you need, from helping you understand what the DASH diet means and the benefits it offers to tips to follow it and detailed recipes and meal plans. All the recipes in this book are easy to cook and hardly take any time in the kitchen. Also, you can eat to your heart's content without worrying about compromising on health or flavor. By following the DASH diet and the recipes in this book, you are eating to get healthier and fitter. All you need to do is simply stock up on the ingredients and items prescribed by the DASH diet and get started. This, coupled with the four-week sample meal plan given in this book, will make your life even easier. Dieting has never been this simple before!

Now that you have all the information needed, what are you waiting for? It is time to start following the protocols of the DASH diet to improve your health. Before you go, could you please do me a small favor? If you loved and enjoyed reading this book or found it helpful se spare a few minutes to leave a review on Amazon.

ink you, and all the best!

References

Bourassa, L. (2019, September 25). DASH diet foods: What to eat & avoid on DASH. Eat This Not That. https://www.eatthis.com/dash-diet-foods-list/

Fries, W. C. (2004, November 4). DASH diet and high blood pressure. WebMD. https://www.webmd.com/hypertension-high-blood-pressure/guide/dash-diet

Hinderliter, A., Babyak, M., Sherwood, A., & Blumenthal, J. (2011, February 1). The DASH diet and insulin sensitivity. Current Hypertension Reports. https://pubmed.ncbi.nlm.nih.gov/21058045/

Ndanuko, R. N., Tapsell, L. C., Charlton, K. E., Neale, E. P., & Batterham, M. J. (2016). Dietary patterns and blood pressure in adults: A systematic review and meta-analysis of randomized controlled trials. Advances in Nutrition, 7(1), 76–89. https://doi.org/10.3945/an.115.009753

Onvani, S., Haghighatdoost, F., & Azadbakht, L. (2015). Dietary approach to stop hypertension (DASH): Diet components may be related to lower prevalence of different kinds of cancer: A review on the related documents. Journal of Research in Medical Sciences: The Official Journal of Isfahan University of Medical Sciences, 20(7), 707–713. https://doi.org/10.4103/1735-1995.166233

Sacks, F. M., Moore, T. J., Appel, L. J., Obarzanek, E., Cutler, J. A., Vollmer, W. M., Vogt, T. M. Karanja, N., Svetkey, L. P., Lin, P.-H., Bray, G. A., & Windhauser, M. M. (1999). A dietary approach to prevent hypertension: A review of the dietary approaches to stop hypertension (DASH) study. Clinical Cardiology, 22(S3), 6–10. https://doi.org/10.1002/clc.4960221506

Salehi-Abargouei, A., Maghsoudi, Z., Shirani, F., & Azadbakht, L. (2013). Effects of dietary approaches to stop hypertension (DASH)-style diet on fatal or nonfatal cardiovascular diseases—Incidence: A systematic review and meta-analysis on observational prospective studies. Nutrition, 29(4), 611–618. https://doi.org/10.1016/j.nut.2012.12.018

Saneei, P., Fallahi, E., Barak, F., Ghasemifard, N., Keshteli, A. H., Yazdannik, A. R., & Esmaillzadeh, A. (2014). Adherence to the DASH diet and prevalence of the metabolic syndrome among Iranian women. European Journal of Nutrition, 54(3), 421–428. https://doi.org/10.1007/s00394-014-0723-y

Satrazemis, E. (2019, September 30). DASH diet guidelines and food lists. Trifecta. https://www.trifectanutrition.com/health/dash-diet-guidelines-and-food-lists

West, H. (2018, October 17). The complete beginner's guide to the DASH diet. Healthline. https://www.healthline.com/nutrition/dash-diet#benefits

Printed in Great Britain
by Amazon

30549729R00064